I0540299

# AUTISM FOR PARENTS

## A COMPREHENSIVE PLAN AND SUPPORT FOR PARENTS TO RECOGNIZE SYMPTOMS, IDENTIFY TRIGGERS, AND ACCESS RESOURCES ACROSS DIFFERENT LIFE STAGES

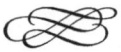

## JAMES R DAVIS

# CONTENTS

# INTRODUCTION

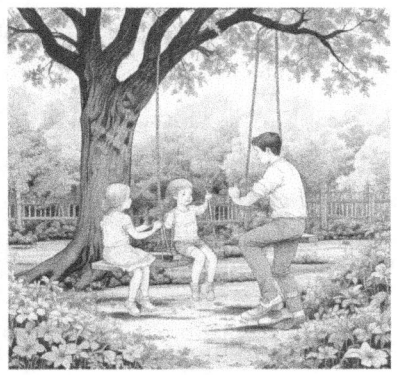

When my grandchild was first diagnosed with Asperger's, I felt a mix of emotions—confusion, concern, but most of all, a deep desire to understand and connect with him on a deeper level. This personal journey has not only taught me about the nuances of Autism Spectrum Disorder (ASD) but has also revealed the profound strength and beauty that lies within these individuals. It is from this personal vantage point that I bring you this book, crafted to guide you, whether you are at the beginning of your journey or looking to deepen your existing knowledge.

The purpose of this book is clear—to provide you with an insightful guide into the world of autism. It is designed to be your companion as you navigate the complexities and joys of understanding and supporting your child with ASD. For those of you who are new to this diagnosis, the book offers foundational knowledge, practical advice, and emotional support. For parents who are further along in this journey, it serves as a resource to gain deeper insights and strategies for continued advocacy and growth.

As a grandfather of a 21-year-old who has thrived with Asperger's, I have walked a path of learning, adaptation, and advocacy. These experiences have not only shaped my grandchild but have transformed me, equipping me with firsthand insights that I am eager to share with you. Through this book, I aim to bridge the gap between scientific research and real-life experiences, providing a narrative that is both informative and deeply human.

This book is unique in its approach, combining the latest scientific research with personal stories and practical advice. It views autism through a lens of strengths and diversity, challenging the deficit-focused narratives that often dominate our discussions about ASD. By highlighting stories of hope and success, the book aims to inspire and uplift you, reinforcing the belief in your child's potential and the diverse ways they can contribute to the world.

The chapters ahead will explore essential topics such as effective communication strategies, navigating educational and healthcare systems, and fostering independence.

Additionally, the book delves into building and leveraging support networks, advocating for change, and actively engaging with the broader autism community. These elements are crucial for both overcoming challenges and celebrating the successes that come with raising a child with ASD.

Given the rapidly evolving landscape of autism research and treatment, this book also touches upon cutting-edge developments and future trends. This ensures that the content not only addresses current needs but also anticipates the questions and challenges of tomorrow.

I encourage you to approach this book with an open heart and mind, ready to learn, accept, and advocate. Together, through shared understanding and collective effort, we can significantly enhance the lives of individuals with autism and their families.

Let us embark on this journey with hope. I believe wholeheartedly in the incredible potential of every child diagnosed with ASD, and I am confident that with the right support and resources, your child, too, can lead a fulfilling and joyful life. Let this book be a stepping stone towards that brighter future.

# UNDERSTANDING AUTISM SPECTRUM DISORDER (ASD)

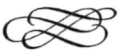

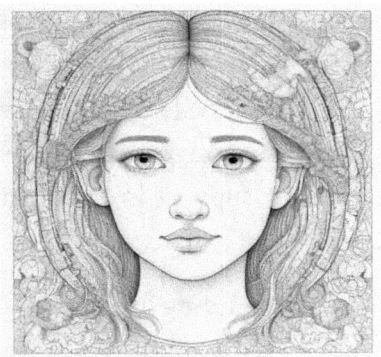

When my grandchild was diagnosed with ASD, a well-meaning friend said, "So, he likes routines and facts, right?" While there's truth in that oversimplification, it barely scratches the surface of what autism encompasses. Autism Spectrum Disorder (ASD) is a complex, multifaceted condition that manifests uniquely in every individual it touches. This chapter aims to unfold the layers of ASD, providing you with a solid understanding of its nuances, the historical evolution of its diagnosis, and why recognizing it early in a child's life can be transformative.

## 1.1 DECODING THE SPECTRUM: AN INTRODUCTION TO AUTISM

Autism Spectrum Disorder (ASD) is a developmental disorder characterized by challenges with social skills, repetitive behaviors, speech and nonverbal communication, as well as by unique strengths and differences. The term "spectrum" in ASD reflects a wide variation in the type and severity of symptoms individuals experience. ASD includes conditions that were previously considered separate — autism, Asperger's syndrome, childhood disintegrative disorder, and an unspecified form of pervasive developmental disorder. Some people with ASD excel in visual skills, music, math, and art. Yet, others might live independently, while some require significant support in their daily lives, underscoring the spectrum's vast range.

Historically, the understanding of autism has undergone significant changes. It was first identified in 1943 by psychiatrist Leo Kanner when he described 11 children who exhibited high intelligence but had difficulties in social interactions and showed a need for sameness. Another turning point came in 1980 when "Infantile Autism" was listed in the Diagnostic and Statistical Manual of Mental Disorders (DSM) for the first time; this helped formalize the diagnostic process and significantly shifted the public and medical perception of the condition. By 2013, all autism disorders were merged under one umbrella diagnosis of ASD in the DSM-5, acknowledging the wide range of symptoms and abilities seen among affected individuals. All this was happening while the prevalence of autism was increasing from 4 to 5 cases per 10,000 people in 1966 to 1 per 100 today. With this said, it is still very uncertain whether this increase is a result of a genuine epidemic , or looser diagnostics, or increased awareness and detection of cases, or as is probably the case, a little bit of all three factors. Undoubtedly however, there is universal agreement that there are some existential and environmental factors at play that are causing this increase. Much effort has taken place in the scientific community to try to find the causes of ASD. All the while many have been debunked, such as childhood vaccinations. Regardless of the causes, at this stage, the purpose of this book is to help you, the parent, identify and cope with the challenges that ASD presents to you and your child so we will continue with this effort.

Understanding the core symptoms of ASD is crucial for early recognition and intervention. The primary symptoms include:

- Social Communication Challenges: Individuals with ASD might find it difficult to maintain eye contact, read body language, or understand the subtleties of conversation. For instance, a child with ASD might not respond to their name being called but will be unusually focused on a particular toy.
- Repetitive Behaviors: Engaging in repetitive behaviors such as rocking, spinning, or the meticulous lining up of objects is common. These actions are often soothing to individuals with ASD.

- Sensory Sensitivities: Many children with ASD have abnormal responses to sensory stimuli. This could mean being greatly bothered by seemingly minor sounds, like the buzzing of a light bulb, or being indifferent to temperatures or pain.

## Importance of Early Identification

Detecting autism early—in the toddler or preschool years—is increasingly seen as a crucial step for effective intervention. Early diagnosis and subsequent interventions can lead to significant improvements in skills and behaviors. This can include better long-term outcomes in language, social functioning, and the ability to adapt to new situations. Interventions can range from behavioral therapy, speech and occupational therapy, to structured teaching and support in school—all tailored to a child's specific needs. Early intervention can tap into the brain's remarkable plasticity during the initial years of life, helping to shape critical social and communication skills.

Moreover, early diagnosis empowers families with knowledge. It provides parents and caregivers the tools and strategies to better support their child's development. Being equipped with this understanding can transform uncertainty into action, creating a pathway toward growth and learning that is informed, compassionate, and responsive to the unique needs of their child with ASD.

In navigating the complexities of ASD, remember, each step taken is a move towards understanding a unique mind. Each child with ASD has a distinct set of capabilities and challenges, and with the right support and intervention, they can reach their full potential. As we explore these nuances, our aim is not just to educate but to foster a community that rises to meet each of its members with empathy, support, and understanding.

## 1.2 BEYOND THE DIAGNOSIS: RECOGNIZING THE DIVERSITY WITHIN ASD

Understanding Autism Spectrum Disorder (ASD) extends beyond recognizing its challenges—it also involves appreciating the distinct strengths and varied abilities that individuals with ASD bring to our world. Often, society focuses predominantly on the difficulties faced by these individuals, overshadowing the remarkable talents many possess. For example, some individuals with ASD have exceptional memory skills, excelling in areas that require attention to detail, such as mathematics, coding, or art. Others might show extraordinary capabilities in music and pitch recognition, or possess an uncanny ability to understand and assemble complex mechanical systems. These strengths can sometimes transform into careers, and more importantly, they can offer avenues for personal satisfaction and self-expression.

Moreover, it's important to recognize that ASD often coexists with other conditions, which can affect how it presents and is managed. Common co-occurring conditions include Attention Deficit Hyperactivity Disorder (ADHD), anxiety disorders, and sensory integration disorders. Each of these can amplify or mask certain aspects of autism, making diagnosis and management a more complex task. For instance, a child with both ASD and ADHD might have heightened difficulties with focus and impulsivity beyond what might be seen in a child with autism alone. Understanding these overlaps is crucial for developing effective treatment plans that address all aspects of a child's development.

Cultural and demographic factors also significantly influence the recognition and management of autism. Across different cultures, symptoms of autism might be interpreted in various ways, affecting how soon, if at all, a child is diagnosed. In some communities, there might be less awareness or acceptance of psychological disorders, leading to delays in seeking or receiving a diagnosis. Additionally, language barriers and socioeconomic factors can limit access to healthcare services, including autism specialists and therapeutic resources, complicating the diagnosis and intervention processes. For families navigating these challenges, finding community support and resources that respect and understand their cultural context is vital.

Personal stories and case studies provide a vivid lens through which to view the diversity within the autism spectrum. Consider the story of a young woman named Maria, who was diagnosed with ASD at the age of four. Growing up, Maria struggled with verbal communication and social interactions. However, her parents and educators noticed her affinity for patterns and numbers. With support, she pursued her interest in mathematics and eventually participated in national math competitions. Maria's story highlights not only the potential for individuals with ASD to achieve remarkable feats in areas of strength but also underscores the importance of personalized support systems that recognize and nurture individual talents.

In exploring these narratives and understanding the broad spectrum of abilities and challenges, we gain a more nuanced perspective of autism. This enriched understanding not only helps in providing better support for individuals with ASD but also celebrates the unique contributions they make to our society. As we continue to learn from each individual's experiences, we enhance our collective ability to foster environments where diversity is not just recognized but is truly valued.

# EARLY DAYS POST-DIAGNOSIS

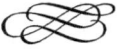

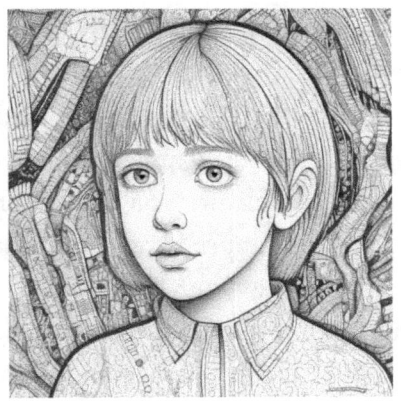

The moment you receive an autism diagnosis for your child, the world may seem to pivot on its axis. It's a point of transformation—not just for your child, but for every member of your family. The initial rush of emotions may cloud your next steps, but gaining clarity on what to do following an autism diagnosis is crucial. This chapter is dedicated to guiding you through these initial steps, providing both the knowledge and tools you need to effectively support your child's development and well-being.

## 2.1 FIRST STEPS AFTER AN AUTISM DIAGNOSIS: PRACTICAL ADVICE

### Understanding the Diagnosis

When the reality of your child's diagnosis settles, the first substantial step is to thoroughly understand what it means. Autism Spectrum Disorder encompasses a broad range of conditions characterized by challenges with social skills, repetitive behaviors, speech, and nonverbal communication, as well as by unique strengths and differences. Each child on the autism spectrum has a distinct set of needs.

It is vital that you, as a parent, fully grasp not just the diagnosis but its specifics concerning your child. This understanding will fundamentally shape how you advocate for and support your child. Request a detailed explanation from your healthcare provider and ensure you leave with a copy of the diagnostic report. This report is not just a document; it's a roadmap that will guide your decisions about therapies, interventions, and supports. It will detail the level of support your child needs, which can range from minimal support for those mildly affected to substantial support for those more significantly challenged.

### Seeking Early Intervention Services

Armed with knowledge and documentation, the next step is to explore early intervention services. Early intervention is crucial as it takes advantage of a child's young brain, which is still forming and is more adaptable to change than at any other time in life. Services typically include speech therapy, occupational therapy, and behavioral therapy, each tailored to meet the specific needs of your child.

To access these services, start by contacting your local early intervention center; you can find these through referrals from your healthcare provider or local health department. The process usually begins with an evaluation of your child's current skills and challenges, which will help to create an intervention plan that targets specific developmental needs. Remember, the goal of early intervention is not just to accelerate development but to equip your child with the skills necessary for as independent a life as possible.

**Setting Up a Support Network**

No one should navigate autism alone—the journey can be profoundly challenging, and a robust support network can be your greatest asset. Start by connecting with local autism support groups; these can be found through social media, hospitals, or autism advocacy organizations. These groups offer an invaluable space to share experiences, advice, and encouragement.

Further, consider engaging with online communities. These platforms can provide support and resources at any time of the day, which is particularly useful during those late-night moments of uncertainty or crisis. Additionally, connecting with broader organizations dedicated to autism can keep you informed about the latest research, workshops, and advocacy opportunities. The emotional and practical support from these networks will be a cornerstone in managing the challenges ahead.

## Educational Rights and School Planning

As your child approaches school age, understanding their educational rights becomes paramount. In the United States, every child with a disability is entitled to a Free Appropriate Public Education (FAPE) under the Individuals with Disabilities Education Act (IDEA). This law ensures that children with disabilities receive an education that is tailored to their individual needs, commonly outlined in an Individualized Education Program (IEP).

To set up an IEP, contact your school's special education department to request an evaluation. An IEP meeting will then be convened, which you should attend as a key member of the team. This plan will detail the specific services your child will receive, the goals for the academic year, and how progress will be measured. Remember, you are an advocate for your child's education—ensure their IEP aligns with their needs and strengths.

## Interactive Element: Resource List

To assist you further, below is a list of resources that can help you navigate the early days post-diagnosis:

- Autism Speaks Toolkits: Offers comprehensive guides for various stages of life with autism.
- CDC's Autism Links and Resources: Provides a broad range of resources, including details on early intervention services.

- Wrightslaw: Offers in-depth information on special education law and advocacy for children with disabilities.

Navigating the initial phase following an autism diagnosis is about laying a strong foundation for your child's growth and your family's journey. With the right understanding, early interventions, support networks, and educational plans in place, you are taking proactive steps toward enhancing your child's development and quality of life. As you move forward, remember that each step you take is building towards a future filled with greater understanding, capability, and hope.

## 2.2 EMOTIONAL SUPPORT FOR FAMILIES POST-DIAGNOSIS

When a child is diagnosed with Autism Spectrum Disorder, the emotional aftermath for the family can be as complex as the condition itself. Parents may traverse a wide spectrum of emotions—from shock and denial to guilt and grief. It's natural to feel overwhelmed as you grapple with what the diagnosis means for your child's future and that of your family. Managing these emotions is not just crucial for your well-being but also for your ability to be the pillar your child needs during this time.

Firstly, acknowledging your feelings is a step towards managing them. Allow yourself to experience and accept these emotions without judgment. Seeking support from partners, friends, or support groups can provide relief and perspective. Stress and guilt, common companions in this journey, can be mitigated through open discussions with others who understand your situation. Techniques such as mindfulness, meditation, or even regular physical activity can significantly alleviate stress. Remember, taking care of yourself is not an indulgence—it's necessary. A healthy you means a more stable environment for your child.

Supporting siblings and other family members is equally important. Brothers and sisters may feel confused, neglected, or even jealous as they witness the sudden shift in family focus towards their sibling with ASD. Honest communication is key—explain what autism is in age-appropriate terms and reassure them of your love and commitment. It's essential to spend quality time with each child, making them feel valued and included. Family activities that include all children can strengthen bonds and promote understanding among siblings.

The dynamics within a family can shift significantly after an autism diagnosis. Roles and responsibilities may evolve, and the stress can strain even the strongest relationships. Couples might find themselves disagreeing more often, especially when it comes to decisions about treatment and education. It's crucial to maintain open lines of communication, share responsibilities, and support each other emotionally. Family therapy can be beneficial in improving communication, resolving conflicts, and adjusting to new family dynamics. Remember, a united family front can provide the strongest support for a child with ASD.

Lastly, consider engaging with professional counseling or therapy. Therapists who specialize in ASD can offer invaluable support in navigating the emotional terrain post-diagnosis. They can provide strategies to cope with grief, tools to manage stress, and techniques to strengthen family relationships. To find a suitable therapist, consult with your healthcare provider or contact local autism organizations for recommendations. Therapy can be a safe space to explore your feelings, develop coping strategies, and ensure your family's emotional resilience.

Navigating the emotional landscape after an autism diagnosis is challenging, yet with the right strategies and supports, families can emerge stronger. Managing personal emotions, supporting each family member, adapting to changes in family dynamics, and seeking professional help are all steps that build a supportive environment for your child. As you move forward, remember that your ability to adapt and grow can foster a nurturing and understanding home, setting the stage for your child's growth and success.

The emotions and adjustments post-diagnosis are just the beginning. As we turn the page to the next chapter, we'll explore strategies for daily communication, which is pivotal in nurturing your child's development and enhancing your family's harmony.

# EVERYDAY STRATEGIES FOR COMMUNICATION

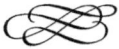

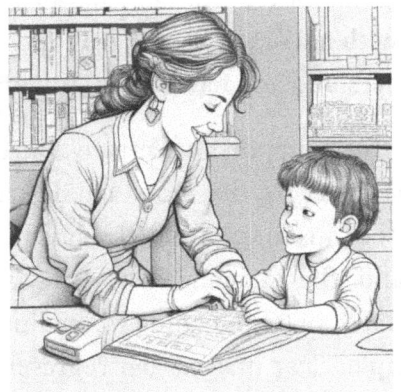

Communication forms the backbone of human interaction and is pivotal in nurturing relationships, yet for a child with Autism Spectrum Disorder (ASD), it can represent a significant challenge. This chapter is dedicated to equipping you with a variety of strategies and tools designed to foster effective communication, bridging the gap between you and your child. By integrating these practices into your daily routine, you can enhance your child's ability to express themselves and interact with the world around them, opening up new avenues for engagement and understanding.

## 3.1 BUILDING A COMMUNICATION BRIDGE: TOOLS AND TECHNIQUES

### Utilizing Visual Supports

Visual supports are an invaluable tool in facilitating communication for children with ASD, particularly for those who are non-verbal or have limited verbal skills. These supports, which include picture cards, visual schedules, and storyboards, leverage the often-strong visual processing abilities of individuals with autism, providing a concrete and consistent way to understand and navigate their world.

To implement visual supports effectively, start by identifying the routines or concepts that your child struggles with or needs to learn. For instance, a visual schedule can help your child understand the sequence of daily activities—from brushing their teeth in the morning to reading a book before bed. Create simple, clear images that represent each activity. These can be hand-drawn or printed pictures. Arrange them in a sequence that mirrors their daily routine, and place the schedule somewhere easily visible. As each activity is completed, encourage your child to remove or mark the corresponding picture. This not only reinforces the concept of sequence but also gives them a sense of accomplishment.

Storyboards can be used to prepare your child for less routine events, such as a visit to the dentist or a family outing. By breaking down the event into a series of steps shown through pictures, you can help reduce anxiety and make unfamiliar situations more predictable.

## Incorporating Technology

In today's digital age, technology offers a plethora of tools that can enhance communication for children with ASD. Tablets and smartphones, equipped with communication apps, can serve as dynamic and interactive communication aids. Apps like Proloquo2Go and Speak for Yourself turn tablets into augmentative and alternative communication (AAC) devices, allowing children to use symbols to construct sentences and communicate their thoughts and needs.

When selecting an app or device, consider your child's motor skills, visual-spatial abilities, and personal interests. It's important to ensure that the interface is intuitive and the content is engaging for your child. Regularly update the content to reflect your child's evolving needs and interests, such as including new vocabulary words that relate to a recently adopted hobby or a new school subject.

Integrating technology should always be a complement to, rather than a replacement for, human interaction. Encourage your child to use their device to communicate with family members and peers, enhancing their social skills and reinforcing the practical use of technology in everyday communication.

## Speech Therapy Techniques

Speech therapy offers a range of techniques that can be adapted for home use to improve your child's verbal communication. Basic exercises can include articulation practice, where you help your child learn how to pronounce certain sounds and words through repetition and correction. This might involve exaggeratedly saying a difficult word and having your child attempt to mimic your articulation.

Language development activities can involve naming objects around the house, describing their actions during play, or organizing simple storytelling sessions. These activities enrich vocabulary and help improve grammar by practicing sentence structure in a natural setting.

Pragmatic language skills, which govern the use of language in social contexts, can be enhanced through role-playing and structured social interactions. Set up scenarios that your child is likely to encounter, such as asking for help in class or sharing toys with a friend, and guide them through the appropriate verbal responses and cues.

**Creating Opportunities for Interaction**

Everyday activities can be transformed into opportunities for communication. Engage your child in interactive games that require taking turns and using specific language, such as board games or simple card games. During these activities, emphasize the use of clear, concise language and encourage your child to articulate their thoughts and choices.

Group activities, whether organized playdates or family gatherings, provide social settings where your child can practice their communication skills. Prior to these events, you can prepare your child by discussing who will be there and what kinds of interactions they might expect. Afterward, discuss how they felt about the interaction and what they might like to do the same or differently next time.

By incorporating these tools and techniques into your daily routine, you actively open up new pathways for your child to express themselves and connect with the world around them. Each strategy not only enhances their ability to communicate but also reinforces your bond, making each interaction a building block for growth and understanding.

## 3.2 UNDERSTANDING AND USING NON-VERBAL COMMUNICATION EFFECTIVELY

Non-verbal communication encompasses a wide array of signals including body language, facial expressions, and eye contact. For children with Autism Spectrum Disorder, who may find verbal communication challenging, these non-verbal cues can both inform and express a great deal. Teaching you to recognize and interpret these signals can significantly improve your interactions with your child. For instance, a child avoiding eye contact might be feeling over-whelmed rather than disinterested, or a certain posture might indicate anxiety. Learning to read these cues involves observing your child in various settings and noting how their non-verbal responses relate to their environment or emotional state.

Moreover, it's equally important for you to use your body language to communicate effectively with your child. Your facial expressions, gestures, and even your tone of voice can provide reassurance, show affection, or convey understanding. For example, a gentle tone and a smile when greeting your child can make them feel welcomed and loved, while a calm demeanor can help soothe them when they're upset. Remember, consistency in your non-verbal communication helps your child understand and predict emotional responses, which is crucial for their sense of security and emotional development.

Sensory sensitivities are another critical aspect of non-verbal communication that needs consideration. Many children with ASD are hypersensitive or hyposensitive to sensory stimuli, which can considerably affect their communication. For instance, a child might cover their ears and look away when in a noisy environment, signaling discomfort. Understanding these responses allows you to adjust their surroundings to better suit their sensory needs, such as reducing background noise or dimming overly bright lights. By creating a sensory-friendly communication environment, you are enabling your child to focus more on the interaction and less on the sensory distractions around them.

Encouraging non-verbal forms of expression such as art, music, or dance can also be incredibly beneficial. These activities offer alternative avenues for children who struggle with traditional forms of communication to express their thoughts and emotions. Art, for instance, can be a powerful tool for self-expression; it allows children to depict their feelings and experiences in a visual format, which can be easier than expressing them verbally. Music and dance can similarly provide emotional outlets and ways to connect with others without words. Engaging your child in these activities not only fosters their creative expression but also boosts their confidence and emotional well-being.

Incorporating an understanding of non-verbal cues and sensory sensitivities, utilizing expressive body language, and encouraging artistic forms of expression can profoundly enrich your communication with your child. These strategies not only enhance understanding but also strengthen your bond, providing your child with the confidence and security they need to express themselves in a world that can often seem overwhelming.

As we close this chapter on communication, we reflect on the critical role that both verbal and non-verbal interactions play in the lives of children with ASD. We've explored practical tools and techniques to enhance these interactions—each fostering connection, understanding, and expression in its unique way. As you continue to apply these strategies, remember that every child is unique, and what works best will often require patience, observation, and adaptation. Moving forward, the next chapter will delve into navigating daily challenges, providing you with strategies to manage and embrace the day-to-day experiences of parenting a child with ASD.

# NAVIGATING DAILY CHALLENGES

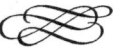

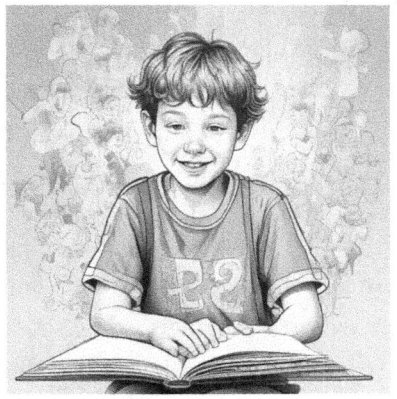

When you step into the world of parenting a child with Autism Spectrum Disorder, each day can seem like a new puzzle—sometimes enchanting, often challenging. Amidst these fluctuations, establishing a consistent daily routine emerges not just as a helpful strategy but as a cornerstone of stability for both you and your child. Routines are the scaffolding that supports your child's understanding of their world, significantly reducing the anxiety that unpredictability can bring. This chapter is devoted to helping you construct and refine these daily routines, making each day a little less uncertain and a lot more manageable.

## 4.1 CREATING CONSISTENT DAILY ROUTINES

### Benefits of Routine for Autistic Children

For children with autism, the world can sometimes feel like an overwhelming place, filled with unexpected events and unpredictable outcomes. Here, routines work like magic—providing a predictable and familiar structure that can significantly alleviate stress. Consistency in daily activities helps children understand what to expect and when to expect it, which can reduce anxiety and prevent many stress-related behaviors. For instance, knowing that after breakfast comes time for schoolwork can help a child transition more smoothly from eating to studying, reducing resistance or meltdowns that stem from sudden changes.

Moreover, routines help in reinforcing a sense of time and sequence, which are often challenging concepts for children on the autism spectrum. Regular schedules reinforce the natural rhythm of the day, from morning routines to bedtime rituals, helping your child navigate the day with greater confidence and less anxiety. This predictability not only supports your child's emotional regulation but also enhances their ability to function independently within the structured framework you provide.

**Steps to Establish a Routine**

Creating a routine that works seamlessly with your child's needs requires thoughtful planning and flexibility. Start by outlining a basic structure for the day, including key activities such as waking up, meal times, therapy sessions, play periods, and bedtime. Each of these should occur at roughly the same time every day to create a predictable pattern. However, it's crucial to allow some flexibility within this structure to accommodate the natural ebb and flow of your child's mood and energy levels. Some days might require more downtime between activities, while others might see your child more receptive to new tasks.

Engage with your child during the planning process. Discuss the schedule with them using simple, clear language, and incorporate their feedback where possible. This might mean choosing between doing homework before or after a snack based on when they feel more energized to focus. Use tools like visual schedules or charts, which can be placed in your child's bedroom or common areas. These visual aids should feature simple, clear images representing each activity, helping your child visualize their day at a glance.

**Involving the Child in Routine Planning**

A child's involvement in creating their daily schedule not only aids in their understanding of it but also empowers them by giving them a sense of control and ownership over their activities. This empowerment can be particularly significant for children with autism, who may often feel that they have little control over their environment. By allowing choices within their routine—such as picking the color of their toothbrush or choosing between two outfits for school —you validate their preferences and encourage decision-making skills.

Discuss the schedule regularly with your child, acknowledging their feelings and preferences. For example, if your child expresses that they feel rushed during morning routines, consider adjusting wake-up times to allow a more relaxed start to the day. This not only helps in fine-tuning the routine to better suit your child's needs but also reinforces their understanding of the sequence of daily activities.

**Tools for Supporting Routines**

To effectively implement and stick to a routine, several tools can be incredibly helpful. Visual schedules, as mentioned, are excellent for children who are visual learners. These can be created using symbols, pictures, or written words, depending on your child's reading skills. Timers are another great tool, especially for activities that your child might resist ending, like playtime. Setting a timer provides a clear signal that an activity is about to end, helping prepare them for the next transition.

Routine charts can also be beneficial, especially when trying to instill new habits or responsibilities, like brushing teeth or packing a school bag. These charts can be used to track progress and can be linked to a reward system to motivate your child. For outings or less frequent activities, consider creating special schedules that outline the steps involved in these events. This can help reduce anxiety about unfamiliar situations and make transitions smoother.

By integrating these strategies and tools into your daily planning, you create a structured yet flexible environment that can significantly ease the daily challenges of parenting a child with ASD. This structured approach not only supports your child's need for predictability but also fosters a sense of security and independence, paving the way for them to engage more confidently with the broader world around them.

## 4.2 MANAGING SENSORY SENSITIVITIES AT HOME

Sensory sensitivities are a prominent aspect of life for many children with Autism Spectrum Disorder (ASD), manifesting in heightened or reduced responses to various stimuli in their environment. These sensitivities can profoundly affect daily activities and behaviors, making ordinary situations like a family dinner or a visit to a grocery store challenging. Understanding and managing these sensitivities at home can create a more supportive environment that caters to the needs of your child.

Sensory sensitivities can vary widely among children with ASD; some may find loud noises overwhelming, while others might not react to sounds that typically garner a response. Similarly, tactile sensitivities can range from an aversion to certain clothing fabrics to being indifferent to temperature extremes. Such variations can influence a child's behavior significantly—what seems like a tantrum might actually be a response to an uncomfortable tag in a shirt or the hum of a fluorescent light. Recognizing these triggers is the first step in creating a sensory-friendly home environment.

One effective strategy is to adjust the home setting to reduce sensory triggers. Start with the lighting—fluorescent lights can be harsh and bothersome; replacing them with LED bulbs that emit a softer, adjustable light can make a significant difference. Consider the use of natural light wherever possible, as it is less harsh and can be soothing. In terms of sound, if your child is sensitive to noise, investing in sound-proofing elements like thick carpets, curtains, and wall panels can help. These modifications not only reduce the volume of external noises but also soften the sounds within the home, creating a calmer environment.

Regarding tactile sensitivities, the choice of furniture and clothing can play a crucial role. Opt for soft, natural fabrics both in clothing and in upholstery. Avoid materials that are scratchy or stiff and choose clothing without tags or with tags that can be easily removed. Furniture should be selected not only for comfort but also for safety—soft corners and cushioned coverings can prevent discomfort and injuries. Each of these adjustments not only eases sensory sensitivities but also enhances the overall comfort of your home for your child.

Implementing a 'sensory diet'—a tailored plan that includes a series of physical activities and experiences designed to engage sensory systems—can be particularly beneficial. This doesn't involve food but rather activities that help your child regulate their response to sensory stimuli. For a child who is overly sensitive to touch, this might include activities like playing with sand or water, which provide gentle, yet varying, tactile feedback. For those sensitive to movement, exercises such as swinging or jumping on a trampoline can help. The key is consistency and incorporation of these activities into your child's daily routine, which can help them process sensory information more effectively and reduce episodes of sensory overload.

In times of sensory overload, having strategies in place to help your child cope is crucial. Recognize the early signs of distress—this might be covering their ears, squinting their eyes, or becoming unusually withdrawn. Once these signs are noticed, guide your child to a predetermined safe space in your home. This should be a quiet, comforting area where they can retreat and regroup. Techniques like deep breathing, listening to calming music, or using weighted blankets can also be effective in alleviating distress. Over time, your child may learn to identify their own signs of sensory overload and seek out their safe space independently, promoting self-regulation.

Managing sensory sensitivities at home requires an understanding of your child's unique needs and a willingness to adapt your environment to meet these needs. Through thoughtful modifications to your home, the implementation of a sensory diet, and strategies to cope with sensory overload, you can create a supportive space that allows your child to feel more comfortable and less overwhelmed by their surroundings. This not only enhances their daily experiences but also contributes to their overall development and well-being.

As we conclude this chapter on managing sensory sensitivities, we've explored various strategies—from modifying the home environment to implementing a sensory diet—that can significantly aid in managing the daily challenges faced by children with ASD. These adaptations not only help in reducing sensory-related distress but also support your child's ability to engage more fully with their environment, paving the way for enhanced learning and interaction. Moving forward, the next chapter will delve into educational insights and advocacy, expanding our focus from the home to the broader realms of school and community, where understanding and support continue to play critical roles in your child's development.

# EDUCATIONAL INSIGHTS AND ADVOCACY

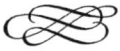

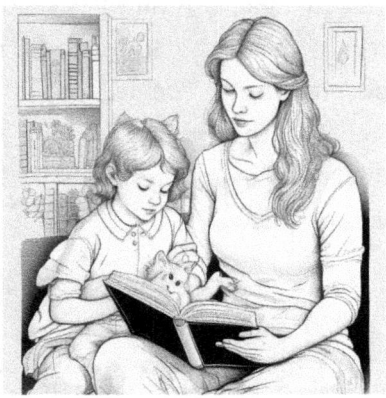

As you navigate the terrain of autism with your child, understanding and engaging with the educational system becomes a pivotal chapter in your ongoing narrative. Particularly, the creation and management of an Individualized Education Program (IEP) stand as one of the most critical advocacy processes you will undertake. This program is not just a document, but a comprehensive plan that outlines specific educational instructions, supports, and services your child requires to thrive in school. The effectiveness of an IEP hinges significantly on your active participation and understanding of its framework, execution, and continual adaptation.

## 5.1 NAVIGATING THE IEP PROCESS: A STEP-BY-STEP GUIDE

**Understanding the IEP**

An Individualized Education Program (IEP) is essentially a blueprint for the education of a child with a disability, recognized and mandated by the Individuals with Disabilities Education Act (IDEA). The IEP outlines specific educational goals, the services needed to achieve these goals, and how progress will be measured. The legal rights encompassed within an IEP ensure that your child receives a tailored education that meets their unique needs in the least restrictive environment possible.

To grasp the nuances of an IEP, it's crucial to familiarize yourself with key terms such as 'Least Restrictive Environment' (LRE), which means that your child should be educated alongside their non-disabled peers to the greatest extent appropriate. Understanding the roles of school personnel involved—from special education teachers to school psychologists—is equally important as these professionals will collaborate with you to develop and implement the IEP. Each member of this team brings a different perspective and expertise, contributing to a more holistic approach to your child's education.

**Preparing for the IEP Meeting**

Preparation is key to a successful IEP meeting. Begin by gathering all necessary documentation related to your child's education and health. This includes medical reports, evaluations from therapists, teacher observations, and your notes on your child's development and challenges. Understanding your child's current performance in school is crucial, so review their latest assessments and report cards. This information will help you set informed, realistic goals for your child's IEP.

Before the meeting, take the time to write down any questions or concerns you have. Think about what accommodations, services, or modifications will support your child's learning and inclusion in school activities. It's helpful to prioritize these needs so you can ensure the most critical points are discussed during the meeting.

**Active Participation in the Meeting**

During the IEP meeting, your role as a parent is pivotal. You are an expert on your child and your insights are invaluable. Communicate openly with the IEP team, sharing your observations and concerns. Be clear about what you feel would best support your child's educational and social development.

Effective communication involves not only expressing your views but also listening to the perspectives of teachers and therapists. Ask clarifying questions to ensure you fully understand the proposed strategies and services. Collaboration is the goal here, with the aim to forge a team that works cohesively to support your child's educational journey.

## Follow-up and Reevaluation

An IEP is not a static document; it's a dynamic plan that should evolve as your child grows and their needs change. Regular monitoring of the IEP's effectiveness is crucial. This includes tracking your child's progress, which should be reported by the school regularly, and ensuring that the agreed-upon services are being provided.

Annual IEP reviews are mandated, but you can request a meeting at any time if you feel adjustments are needed. If your child is not meeting their educational goals, discuss what changes might be necessary with the IEP team. This could involve introducing new services, adjusting goals, or even reevaluating the educational placement. Keeping thorough records of your child's progress and any communications with school staff is important and can be invaluable during these discussions.

## Interactive Element: IEP Checklist

To aid in your preparation and ensure you cover all necessary bases, below is a checklist for the IEP process:

- Documentation: Gather all medical reports, therapist evaluations, and school reports.
- Goals: List specific short-term and long-term educational goals for your child.

- Questions: Write down any questions or concerns about your child's education.
- Priorities: Determine what accommodations or services are most crucial for your child.
- Follow-up: Schedule dates for checking in on your child's progress post-IEP meeting.

Navigating the IEP process effectively sets a strong foundation for your child's educational path. It is a significant advocacy tool that, when utilized correctly, can greatly enhance your child's ability to succeed and flourish in the educational setting. As you step into this role, remember that your involvement and voice are integral to shaping the educational experiences and outcomes for your child.

## 5.2 ENSURING INCLUSIVE EDUCATION: STRATEGIES FOR PARENTS

Inclusive education is founded on the principle that all children, regardless of their abilities or disabilities, have the right to be educated together in the least restrictive environment. This educational approach not only benefits children with Autism Spectrum Disorder (ASD) by providing them with opportunities to learn alongside their neurotypical peers but also enriches the educational experience of all students by fostering a culture of diversity and mutual respect. The legal backing for inclusive education primarily comes from the Individuals with Disabilities Education Act (IDEA), which supports the rights of students to receive an appropriate education in the least restrictive environment possible.

Building positive relationships with educators and school staff is crucial in navigating the path toward inclusive education. As a parent, your engagement with teachers, aides, and administrators sets the foundation for collaborative partnerships. Start by clearly communicating your child's needs and strengths, and express your desire for inclusion. Regular meetings and open lines of communication help ensure that everyone involved is aligned with your child's educational goals. When advocating for necessary supports and accommodations, approach discussions with respect and a willingness to listen, which can facilitate more productive conversations and solutions.

Moreover, the integration of specific educational tools and technologies can significantly enhance the inclusivity of the classroom for students with autism. Tools such as text-to-speech software, visual schedules, and sensory integration items can be vital in supporting your child's learning and participation. Advocating for the use of these tools involves demonstrating their benefits not only for your child but for the entire classroom, as many of these tools can improve the overall learning environment. For instance, visual aids can help clarify instructions and routines for all students, not just those with ASD.

Community and peer engagement plays a transformative role in promoting an inclusive educational environment. Encouraging positive interactions between your child and their peers is essential. This can be facilitated through joint activities that play to the strengths of children with ASD, such as structured group projects or technology-based tasks where these students often excel. Additionally, educating peers about autism can cultivate an atmosphere of understanding and acceptance. Programs that involve peer mentoring, buddy systems, and inclusive sports and clubs are also effective in enhancing social integration. These initiatives not only help demystify autism for other students but also highlight the shared interests and humanity of all children, regardless of their developmental differences.

Navigating the landscape of inclusive education requires a proactive and informed approach, but the benefits for your child and their peers are profound. By fostering partnerships with educators, advocating for effective tools and accommodations, and promoting positive peer interactions, you can help create an educational environment where diversity is valued and all children are given the opportunity to thrive.

As this chapter concludes, we reflect on the pivotal role that inclusive education plays in the broader spectrum of your child's development and societal integration. The strategies outlined here are designed not just to support your child but to enhance the educational landscape in a way that respects and celebrates diversity. Moving forward, the next chapter will delve into the dynamics of social skills and interaction, exploring how these critical elements influence your child's ability to navigate their social world.

# SOCIAL SKILLS AND INTERACTION

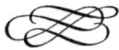

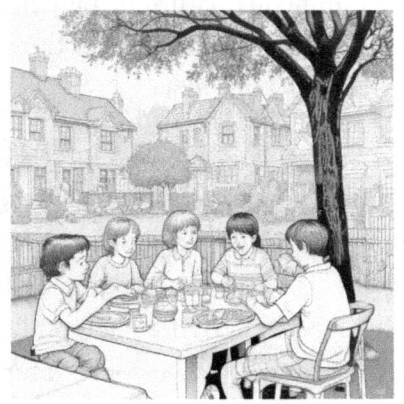

Navigating the complexities of social interactions can be a significant challenge for children with Autism Spectrum Disorder (ASD), yet mastering these skills is crucial for their personal and social development. This chapter delves into the nuanced role of play in enhancing social skills, offering strategies and insights into making each playful moment a stepping stone towards building better social interactions. Here, we explore how the structured yet flexible nature of play can be harnessed to teach essential social skills in an engaging, supportive, and practical manner.

## 6.1 TEACHING SOCIAL SKILLS THROUGH PLAY

**Role of Play in Social Development**

Play is the language of childhood. Through play, children explore the world, learn new skills, and connect with others. For children with autism, play acts not just as a source of joy, but as a critical educational tool that teaches them how to communicate, share, take turns, and express themselves. The structured yet spontaneous nature of play helps in breaking down the complexities of social interactions into manageable, enjoyable learning experiences.

In the realm of play, each action and interaction serves as a live lesson in social dynamics. For instance, when a child passes a ball to another, they are not just engaging in physical activity, but are also learning the give-and-take nature of social relationships. Such activities help children with ASD understand the cause and effect of social interactions, recognize emotional expressions, and develop the patience required to listen and respond to another person's actions or words.

Moreover, play provides a safe space for children with ASD to experiment with different social behaviors and roles. Through role-play, children can explore various social scenarios and their appropriate responses without the fear of real-world repercussions. This can significantly boost their confidence and comfort level in social settings.

**Choosing Appropriate Toys and Games**

Selecting the right toys and games is crucial in fostering an environment conducive to social learning. The key is to choose items that match the child's developmental level and interests, and that inherently encourage interaction with others. For example, simple board games that require turn-taking can teach children the importance of waiting and the joy of participating cooperatively.

Toys that stimulate shared interests, such as building blocks for children who like constructing, can encourage them to engage with peers who have similar preferences. This not only keeps them engaged but also provides common ground for interaction. When choosing toys, consider those that are versatile and open-ended; these allow children to innovate and decide how to use them, which can lead to more natural opportunities for interaction and cooperation with others.

**Structured Play Activities**

Structured play activities are designed with clear goals and guidelines that help direct the child's engagement and learning. These activities can be particularly beneficial for children with ASD, who may thrive in environments where expectations are clear and consistent. Examples of structured play activities include role-playing games, cooperative board games, and team sports, all of which require children to work together toward a common goal.

Role-playing games, for instance, allow children to act out different scenarios—like a visit to the doctor or a day at school. These games can help children practice appropriate social behaviors and verbal exchanges. Cooperative board games that require players to work together to achieve a win can teach the value of teamwork and collective problem-solving. Team sports, even those adapted to be more inclusive and less competitive, can instill concepts of team dynamics, effort, and sportsmanship.

**Parental Involvement and Facilitation**

Your role as a parent in facilitating play is instrumental. By participating in play, you can guide your child through the complexities of social interactions and help them decode the subtle cues and rules that govern these exchanges. It's about striking a balance—being involved enough to provide guidance and security, but also stepping back to let your child explore and interact independently.

One effective strategy is to narrate the play's social cues out loud. For example, if your child is playing with another child who seems upset, you might say, "It looks like he's sad because his tower fell down. Maybe we can help him build it again?" This not only teaches empathy but also suggests appropriate social responses. Additionally, setting up playdates with peers who have similar interests or developmental levels can provide your child with more opportunities to practice social skills in a controlled and familiar environment. These sessions can be short to ensure they end on a positive note, gradually increasing in duration as your child becomes more comfortable and skilled in navigating social interactions.

Through these methods, play becomes more than just a source of fun; it transforms into a dynamic classroom where social skills are developed, refined, and mastered. As you integrate these strategies into your daily interactions with your child, remember that each child's progress is unique. Patience and persistence are key in helping your child navigate the intricate dance of social interactions.

## 6.2 FACILITATING FRIENDSHIPS: ENCOURAGING POSITIVE SOCIAL INTERACTIONS

Navigating the social world can be complex for children with Autism Spectrum Disorder (ASD), but fostering meaningful friendships is crucial for their social and emotional development. As parents, actively creating and leveraging social opportunities can pave the way for these valuable interactions. Initiating playdates is one of the most direct methods to encourage socialization. These should be planned with careful consideration, ideally involving peers who share similar interests or are understanding and patient. This could mean setting up play sessions with classmates or neighbors who your child feels comfortable with or who have shown a friendly interest in them. Additionally, seeking out local clubs or groups that align with your child's hobbies or passions—be it a book club, a gardening group, or a sports team—can provide a natural setting for social interactions within a structured environment that feels less intimidating.

Participation in community activities, such as local fairs, children's workshops, or charity events, can also widen your child's social circle. These activities offer diverse settings where your child can meet others outside of the usual school environment, which can be particularly beneficial. When attending these events, a familiar routine or a few practiced social scripts can help your child feel more at ease. It's also helpful to brief any facilitators or involved adults about your child's needs and strengths, ensuring they facilitate inclusion in group activities.

Teaching social etiquette and rules form the bedrock of how children interact with each other. Begin by modeling basic social rules at home, such as taking turns during conversations, using polite expressions, and respecting personal space. Role-playing can be an effective tool here. For instance, you could set up a scenario where one person acts out asking for a turn with a toy, helping your child understand how to express their needs and respond to others' requests. Regular practice through role-playing can help solidify these concepts, making real-world application less daunting for your child.

Addressing and preparing for social challenges is equally important. Children with ASD might face situations of rejection or conflict, which can be disheartening and confusing. Preparing your child for such possibilities involves discussing potential scenarios they might encounter and role-playing appropriate responses. For example, practicing what to do or say if a peer does not want to share a toy or if a misunderstanding occurs during a game. Teaching resilience in these situations is crucial; this could involve helping your child understand that not every social interaction will go as expected, and that's okay. Encouraging them to express their feelings about social interactions can also provide you with insights into their personal challenges and successes.

Moreover, fostering an environment of peer support and advocacy is essential. This can be facilitated by involving classmates and friends in the learning process about autism. Workshops or presentations that explain ASD in child-friendly language can enhance peers' understanding and foster a supportive school environment. Encouraging inclusive interactions not just at school but also in social and community settings can broaden the circle of support for your child, helping them feel accepted and valued.

In this interconnected world, fostering friendships for a child with ASD involves more than just facilitating social interactions. It's about creating a supportive network, teaching the nuances of social communication, and preparing for the hurdles along the way. Through these efforts, your child can experience the joys and lessons that come with building and maintaining friendships.

As this chapter concludes, we reflect on the strategies discussed that not only aim to improve your child's social skills but also enhance their overall ability to form and sustain friendships. From structuring playdates to teaching social etiquette and preparing for social challenges, each element contributes to a richer, more supportive social experience for your child. Moving forward, the next chapter will explore behavioral insights and interventions, further enhancing our understanding of how to support children with ASD in more complex social and behavioral scenarios.

# BEHAVIORAL INSIGHTS AND INTERVENTIONS

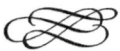

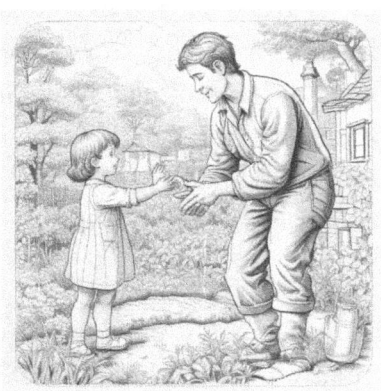

Navigating the behavioral landscape of a child with Autism Spectrum Disorder (ASD) can often feel like deciphering a complex code where each behavior holds a myriad of meanings and messages. This chapter aims to equip you with the insights and tools necessary to understand and effectively respond to these behavioral challenges. By delving into the reasons behind certain behaviors, you can better support your child in managing and overcoming these challenges, ultimately leading to a more harmonious daily life for your entire family.

## 7.1 UNDERSTANDING THE REASONS BEHIND BEHAVIORAL CHALLENGES

### Identifying Common Behavioral Challenges

Children with autism may exhibit a range of behaviors that can be perplexing and, at times, challenging to manage. These behaviors often serve as a manifestation of the internal and external struggles they face. Common behaviors include tantrums, aggression, and self-injurious behavior, each varying widely in frequency, form, and intensity. For instance, while tantrums in typically developing peers might often stem from unmet desires or fatigue, in children with ASD, these outbursts can also arise from overwhelming sensory environments or frustrations due to communication difficulties.

Aggression—whether verbal or physical—can similarly be a product of the intense stress or anxiety a child with autism experiences daily. It's crucial to understand that these behaviors are not acts of defiance but rather involuntary responses to an array of overwhelming stimuli or emotions they cannot otherwise articulate. Self-injurious behaviors, such as head-banging or hand-biting, are particularly distressing for parents to witness. These behaviors often indicate a high level of distress or an attempt to communicate physical pain or discomfort, providing critical clues into the child's state of mind and physical well-being.

## Underlying Causes of Behavioral Issues

The root causes of behavioral challenges in children with autism are as diverse as the spectrum itself. A primary factor is the inherent difficulty they have in communicating needs and desires. When a child cannot verbally express their discomfort, hunger, or need for a break, frustration mounts, often culminating in a behavioral episode. Sensory sensitivities also play a significant role; for many children with ASD, the world is a barrage of sensory information that they cannot filter out, leading to sensory overload and subsequent behavioral outbursts.

Environmental factors such as unexpected changes in routine, noisy settings, or unfamiliar places can further exacerbate these challenges. Each of these elements can disrupt the child's sense of security and predictability, leading to anxiety and stress, which may be expressed through behaviors that are seen as challenging.

## The Role of Anxiety and Stress

Anxiety and stress are frequent companions for many children with autism and can significantly influence their behavior. Understanding the signs of anxiety in your child is vital for early intervention. Signs can include an increase in repetitive behaviors, disruptions in sleep patterns, or sudden changes in mood. Anxiety often serves as a precursor to more intense behavioral episodes; hence, identifying and managing anxiety can help in preventing these episodes.

For instance, if a child becomes particularly clingy or starts to exhibit increase in body rocking, these could be indicators of rising anxiety. Such behaviors may escalate to aggression or tantrums if the anxiety is not addressed. Teaching your child coping mechanisms such as deep breathing, providing a quiet space, or using sensory tools like weighted blankets can help manage their anxiety and reduce the occurrence of disruptive behaviors.

**Assessment Tools and Techniques**

To effectively address and manage behaviors, a thorough and ongoing assessment is essential. Functional Behavior Assessments (FBA) are widely used by professionals to understand the context of behavior in children with autism. This assessment involves observing the child in different settings and at different times to identify specific triggers and consequences that maintain the behavior.

The FBA seeks to answer important questions: What happens before the behavior that might trigger it? What consequences are maintaining the behavior? Understanding these can help in developing strategies that address the root causes rather than merely the symptoms. For example, if a child learns that screaming gets them out of doing tasks they find difficult, they may continue to use this behavior to avoid similar situations in the future. In such cases, alternative, more appropriate behaviors that can achieve the same result for the child need to be taught and reinforced.

**Interactive Element: Reflective Journaling Prompt**

To deepen your understanding and application of the concepts discussed, consider maintaining a reflective journal. Here's a prompt to get you started: Reflect on a recent behavioral challenge you encountered with your child. Based on what you've learned about identifying triggers and underlying causes, can you hypothesize what might have led to this behavior? How can this insight shape your approach to similar situations in the future?

By understanding the "why" behind your child's behaviors, you are better equipped to meet their needs and guide them towards more positive and effective ways of interacting with their world. This not only improves their quality of life but also enhances the well-being of your family as a whole. As we continue to explore these behavioral interventions, remember that each child with ASD is unique, and what works for one may not work for another. Patience, persistence, and continued learning are your best tools as you navigate this complex but ultimately rewarding landscape.

## 7.2 EFFECTIVE AND COMPASSIONATE BEHAVIORAL MANAGEMENT TECHNIQUES

Addressing the behavioral challenges of a child with Autism Spectrum Disorder (ASD) demands a compassionate, proactive approach that seeks to understand and meet underlying needs, rather than merely controlling outward actions. Positive Behavior Support (PBS) is a framework designed for this purpose. It focuses on redesigning environments and changing lifestyle factors to improve overall behavior. At its core, PBS is about understanding why certain behaviors occur and addressing those causes with positive, supportive interventions rather than punitive measures.

PBS begins by identifying the specific needs that drive undesirable behaviors. For instance, if a child finds a particular classroom setting overwhelming, leading to disruptive behavior, the solution might involve adjusting the sensory inputs in that environment, such as reducing noise levels or altering lighting. This proactive approach not only helps in managing the behavior but also supports the child's well-being and development. The goal is to create environments that inherently support positive behaviors, making it easier for the child to engage and learn effectively.

Fostering desirable behaviors in children with ASD often hinges on the consistent application of positive reinforcement. This technique involves identifying a behavior you want to encourage and then providing a positive stimulus immediately after the behavior occurs, thereby increasing the likelihood of the behavior recurring. Reinforcements can vary widely depending on what motivates your child; they could be verbal praises, a favorite snack, tokens, or extra time with a preferred activity. The key is consistency and immediacy, ensuring that the reinforcement directly follows the desirable behavior, making the connection clear and understandable for the child.

For instance, if a child completes a difficult task without outbursts, immediately recognizing this achievement with a preferred reward reinforces the behavior. Over time, these positive reinforcements help in building more adaptive behaviors and reducing reliance on behaviors that challenge. It's vital, however, to tailor these reinforcements to align with your child's preferences and needs, ensuring they are meaningful and motivating for them.

Managing and reducing problematic behaviors involves setting clear, consistent boundaries in a compassionate manner. Children with ASD often benefit from knowing exactly what is expected of them and the consequences of their actions. Establishing these boundaries with clear, simple language and visual supports can help them understand and adhere to these guidelines. When problematic behaviors occur, it's crucial to employ de-escalation techniques before these behaviors escalate. Techniques might include distraction, offering a calming activity, or moving to a quieter space. These strategies help in managing the situation safely and compassionately, reducing stress for both you and your child.

Teaching alternative behaviors is also essential. This involves identifying the need that a problematic behavior is fulfilling and then teaching your child a more appropriate behavior that achieves the same result. For example, if a child tends to scream for attention, teaching them to tap a bell or raise a hand as a signal can be an effective alternative. This method not only addresses the immediate behavior but also equips the child with tools for better communication in the future.

Collaboration with therapists, educators, and other professionals plays a critical role in managing behavioral challenges effectively. These professionals bring a wealth of knowledge and experience and can offer insights and strategies that complement your efforts at home. Regularly communicating with your child's educational and therapeutic teams ensures that everyone is aligned on the strategies being used and can adapt them as necessary to meet your child's evolving needs. This consistent, unified approach helps reinforce learning and behavior management across different settings, providing your child with a cohesive support system.

Effective behavioral management is not just about reducing challenges; it's about enhancing your child's ability to participate fully and joyfully in life. By using Positive Behavior Support, consistently applying positive reinforcements, managing behaviors compassionately, and collaborating with professionals, you create a supportive framework that empowers your child to thrive.

As we conclude this exploration of behavioral insights and interventions, we've equipped ourselves with strategies not only for managing challenges but for fostering an environment that supports positive development. In the next chapter, we'll shift our focus from behavior to the role of technology in autism, exploring how various tools and apps can support learning and communication for children with ASD.

# THE ROLE OF TECHNOLOGY IN AUTISM

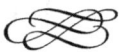

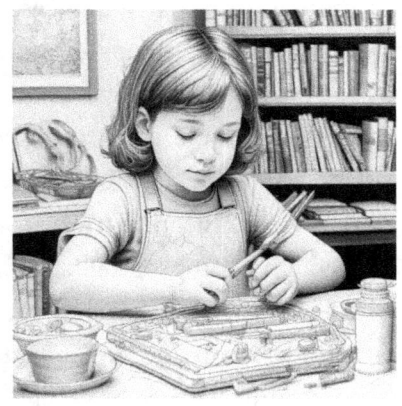

In the vast and ever-evolving landscape of autism support, technology stands out as a beacon of possibility and progress. For many children with Autism Spectrum Disorder (ASD), communicating their thoughts and feelings can be a labyrinthine challenge—one where traditional paths prove inadequate. However, the advent of assistive communication technologies has opened new doors, offering these children a voice through innovative tools that transcend conventional limitations. This chapter delves into how these technological aids can transform the lives of those with significant communication hurdles, illustrating a future where every child has the tools to express themselves freely and fully.

## 8.1 ASSISTIVE TECHNOLOGIES: TOOLS FOR ENHANCING COMMUNICATION

**Overview of Assistive Communication Technologies**

The spectrum of assistive communication technologies available today is broad, comprising Augmentative and Alternative Communication (AAC) devices, speech-generating devices, and various digital apps designed to aid those who are non-verbal or have significant speech challenges. AAC devices range from simple picture boards to sophisticated systems that generate speech through text or symbols. Speech-generating devices, often portable, allow users to input text either through typing or selection, which is then converted into spoken words. Digital apps, accessible on tablets and smartphones, provide flexible and interactive platforms for communication, offering features like customizable pictograms and voice output.

These technologies are not just tools; they are gateways to independence and self-expression for individuals with autism. For a child who has never spoken a word, being able to express a need, a thought, or a feeling using an AAC device can be profoundly liberating. The impact of these technologies extends beyond the user, affecting family dynamics, educational opportunities, and social interactions. They provide a means for clearer understanding and interaction, reducing frustrations and misunderstandings that can occur from communication difficulties.

## Customizing Technologies to Fit Individual Needs

The key to effectively utilizing assistive communication technologies lies in their customization. No two children with autism are the same; thus, the technology must be tailored to meet the unique communication needs of each child. This process begins with a thorough assessment of the child's current communication abilities, which can be conducted by a qualified speech-language pathologist. This assessment will help determine the most suitable type of assistive technology based on the child's motor skills, cognitive levels, and personal preferences.

Selecting the right device or app is just the beginning. Customization might involve programming specific phrases that are relevant to the child's daily life, or adjusting the settings to align with their sensory preferences, such as the volume of voice output or the sensitivity of touch screens. Ongoing adjustments are often necessary as the child's skills and needs evolve over time, making regular collaboration with speech therapists and educators a crucial part of the process.

## Training and Implementation

Introducing a child to new technology requires patience and structured training. The goal is to make the technology a natural part of the child's daily communication. Initially, this might involve short, focused sessions where the child learns to associate specific buttons or symbols with their corresponding outputs. Over time, these sessions can expand to incorporate more complex commands and concepts.

Parental involvement is vital in this training process. By integrating the use of the technology into everyday activities, parents can reinforce learning and encourage consistent use. For example, during mealtime, a child can be prompted to use their device to request specific foods or express satisfaction. Similarly, integrating the technology into classroom activities can enhance the learning experience and promote inclusion among peers.

## Benefits and Limitations

The benefits of using assistive communication technologies are manifold. They provide a voice to those who might otherwise be unable to express themselves, fostering greater independence and self-esteem. The ability to communicate needs, preferences, and emotions can significantly improve the quality of life for a child with ASD, reducing behavior problems that stem from frustration and misunderstandings.

However, it's important to acknowledge the limitations of these technologies. Dependence on devices for communication can sometimes inhibit the development of verbal skills in some children. Therefore, it is crucial to use these tools as part of a broader, balanced approach that includes speech therapy and other communication strategies. Moreover, the high cost of some advanced devices can be a barrier for many families, although funding support may be available through educational programs or health insurance.

**Interactive Element: Checklist for Assessing Assistive Technology Needs**

To assist you in starting the process of selecting and implementing assistive communication technologies, consider the following checklist:

- Assessment of Communication Skills: Has your child been evaluated by a speech-language pathologist to determine their current communication abilities?
- Goals for Communication: What are your specific goals for your child's communication development? How can technology help achieve these goals?
- Research Available Technologies: Have you researched the different types of AAC devices and digital apps available? Consider factors such as ease of use, customization options, and portability.
- Trial Periods: Can you arrange trial periods for devices to determine which one your child adapts to best?
- Training Opportunities: Are there training sessions available for both you and your child to learn how to effectively use the technology?
- Integration into Daily Routines: How can you integrate the use of the technology into your daily routines to maximize its effectiveness?
- Feedback and Adjustments: How will you track the effectiveness of the technology, and what process will you follow to make necessary adjustments?

By thoroughly exploring these areas, you can make informed decisions that enhance your child's ability to communicate and interact with the world around them. This proactive approach not only maximizes the benefits of assistive technologies but also ensures that they serve as valuable tools in your child's developmental journey, fostering a sense of connection and understanding that every child deserves.

## 8.2 EDUCATIONAL APPS AND GAMES FOR LEARNING ENHANCEMENT

In the dynamic landscape of educational technology, a myriad of apps and games have been specifically designed to cater to the unique learning needs of children with Autism Spectrum Disorder (ASD). These digital tools are not just about engagement; they are about opening new doors to learning that traditional methods might not address as effectively. Selecting the right app involves several crucial considerations. The app must captivate the child's interest, ensuring it is engaging enough to keep them focused and involved. Simplicity is key; the interface should be intuitive, avoiding complex navigation that could frustrate a child with ASD. It's also essential that the app aligns well with the child's educational goals—whether it's improving language skills, enhancing social interactions, or mastering daily routines. Additionally, the ability to track the child's progress within the app allows for ongoing assessment of its effectiveness and the child's engagement levels.

Among the plethora of options available, some apps have stood out for their proven efficacy and user-friendly design. For language development, the "Proloquo2Go" app offers a robust augmentative communication solution that helps children who are non-verbal or have limited speech to communicate their thoughts and needs. Its customizable features allow for tailoring vocabulary to the child's daily life, making communication more relevant and straightforward. For enhancing social skills, "Social Stories" provides a platform where children can visualize and rehearse social interactions in a controlled, digital environment. This app helps in breaking down social encounters into manageable parts, making them easier to understand and execute. To assist with daily routines, "Choiceworks" is an excellent tool that helps children manage their daily schedules, understand their feelings, and improve their waiting skills through the use of clear visuals and structured timelines. For basic academic skills, "Endless Alphabet" sets itself apart by turning learning into a fun activity with its engaging, interactive puzzles that teach letter recognition and vocabulary.

Integrating these apps into a child's learning plan should be a thoughtful, strategic process. These digital tools are best used as supplements to traditional teaching methods or therapy sessions, reinforcing the skills being taught. For instance, if a child is learning new vocabulary words during speech therapy, using an app like "Endless Alphabet" at home can reinforce this learning in a playful, interactive way. Similarly, social skills practiced in a therapy setting can be rehearsed using "Social Stories", providing a safe space for the child to practice and gain confidence. The key is consistency; regular use of these apps can help solidify the skills being learned and provide the repetition that is often crucial for children with ASD.

Monitoring how a child interacts with educational apps is crucial. Observing not just the time they spend but how they engage with the app provides insights into its suitability and effectiveness. Are they frustrated or disinterested, or do they seem enthusiastic and focused? Adjustments might be necessary based on these observations. For instance, if an app is too challenging or too easy, it might not hold the child's interest long-term. Regularly consulting with educational professionals who understand your child's specific needs can also provide guidance on how best to use these digital tools. These experts can offer advice on other apps or strategies that might be better suited to your child's evolving educational requirements.

As technology continues to advance, the potential for educational apps and games to support the learning needs of children with ASD expands. By carefully selecting, integrating, and monitoring these digital tools, you can significantly enhance your child's learning experience, providing them with the skills they need to navigate their world more effectively.

In summarizing, this chapter explored the critical role of technology in enhancing the educational journey of children with Autism Spectrum Disorder. From selecting appropriate apps to integrating them into learning plans, each step is aimed at maximizing the benefits these digital tools offer. As we move forward, the next chapter will delve into the importance of sensory-friendly environments, building on our understanding of how tailored adjustments in daily settings can further support the developmental needs of children with ASD.

# HEALTH AND AUTISM

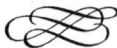

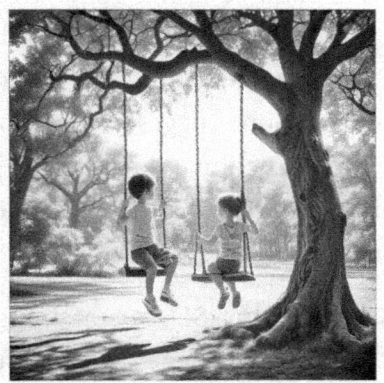

Navigating the intricate landscape of health within the context of Autism Spectrum Disorder (ASD) presents a unique set of challenges and opportunities. The connection between physical health and behavioral manifestations is profound, with dietary considerations playing a pivotal role. As you strive to support your child's well-being, understanding the nuances of how their body reacts to different foods, and how their digestive health influences their behavior and cognitive functions, becomes essential. This chapter delves into the crucial aspects of dietary considerations, aiming to provide you with the knowledge and tools needed to optimize your child's health and, consequently, their quality of life.

## 9.1 DIETARY CONSIDERATIONS AND AUTISM

### Understanding the Gut-Brain Connection

Recent studies have illuminated the significant impact of the gut-brain axis on autism, revealing that the digestive system does more than process food—it also plays a key role in regulating emotions and cognitive functions. The gut-brain axis refers to the biochemical signaling that takes place between the gastrointestinal tract and the central nervous system. This connection suggests that the gut's health directly affects brain function, which is why gastrointestinal issues can sometimes manifest as behavioral changes in children with autism.

For many children with ASD, maintaining balanced gut health is a continual challenge, which can significantly impact their behavior and ability to focus. Issues such as increased intestinal permeability (often referred to as 'leaky gut') and imbalances in gut microbiota could exacerbate some symptoms of autism. Addressing these gastrointestinal issues through dietary adjustments can lead to noticeable improvements in behavior and cognitive functions, making the understanding of this connection a critical component of managing ASD.

## Common Dietary Challenges

Children with ASD often face various dietary challenges, including food sensitivities and selective eating patterns, which can complicate their nutritional intake. Common sensitivities include reactions to gluten, casein (a protein found in milk and dairy products), soy, and certain additives, which can manifest as behavioral disruptions, skin rashes, or gastrointestinal discomfort. Selective eating patterns may also arise from sensory sensitivities, where the texture, color, or smell of certain foods can be overwhelming, leading to a limited diet that may lack essential nutrients.

Early recognition of these dietary challenges is crucial. Observing your child's reaction to certain foods and maintaining a detailed food diary can help identify specific triggers. This record-keeping should include details about what was eaten, the quantities, and any subsequent reactions, both physical and behavioral. Sharing this information with healthcare professionals can aid in developing a tailored dietary plan that addresses these sensitivities and meets nutritional needs.

### Implementing a Gluten-Free and Casein-Free Diet

One dietary approach that has gained attention among parents of children with autism is the gluten-free and casein-free (GFCF) diet. This diet involves eliminating all sources of gluten and casein, which some studies suggest could reduce symptoms of autism, particularly in areas of social interaction and verbal communication. The theory behind this diet is based on the premise that children with ASD may have increased sensitivity or an inability to properly digest gluten and casein, potentially leading to an exacerbation of symptoms.

Implementing a GFCF diet requires careful planning and commitment. Start by educating yourself about which foods contain gluten and casein—gluten is found in wheat, barley, and rye, while casein is present in milk and dairy products. Reading food labels becomes a necessity; look for terms like 'wheat flour,' 'barley malt,' or 'milk solids.' Opt for naturally gluten-free and casein-free foods such as fruits, vegetables, meats, and most dairy-free alternatives. Planning meals can be challenging initially, but numerous resources and recipes are available to help you navigate this diet. Always consult with a dietitian to ensure that your child's nutritional needs are being met, particularly in terms of calcium and vitamin D, which are common in dairy products.

### Assessing Nutritional Needs and Supplements

Due to the restrictive nature of their diets, children with autism might be at risk of certain nutritional deficiencies. A comprehensive nutritional assessment conducted by a healthcare professional can determine if your child is receiving adequate vitamins, minerals, and other essential nutrients. Based on this assessment, supplementation may be necessary to achieve nutritional balance.

Common supplements for children on restrictive diets include calcium, vitamin D, omega-3 fatty acids, and probiotics, each playing a unique role in supporting overall health. For instance, omega-3 fatty acids are critical for brain development and function, while probiotics can aid in maintaining gut health. When choosing supplements, it's essential to opt for high-quality products and to discuss appropriate dosages with your healthcare provider to ensure safety and efficacy.

Navigating the dietary needs of a child with ASD can be complex but understanding and addressing these needs plays a crucial role in supporting their overall health and well-being. By informed management of their diet, you can help alleviate some behavioral issues associated with ASD, contributing to a better quality of life for your child.

## 9.2 EXERCISE AND PHYSICAL ACTIVITIES FOR CHILDREN WITH AUTISM

The importance of regular physical activity extends beyond the general health benefits it offers; for children with Autism Spectrum Disorder (ASD), it can be a pivotal element in enhancing their overall well-being and development. Engaging in appropriate physical activities can significantly improve motor skills, which are often delayed in children with autism. These activities help refine their coordination and muscle control, providing a foundation for more complex movements and skills. Furthermore, exercise serves as a natural stress reliever; physical activities can help reduce anxiety levels and improve mood by releasing endorphins, known as the body's natural feel-good neurotransmitters. Social skills, too, can see marked improvement through structured group exercises, where children learn to follow rules, take turns, and engage in teamwork.

Selecting the right type of physical activities for your child involves understanding their unique preferences, abilities, and sensory processing needs. Some children might find great joy and less sensory conflict in individual sports like swimming or horseback riding, which allow for a calming, rhythmic experience with minimal unexpected tactile feedback. Swimming, in particular, is often therapeutic for children with autism as the water provides a comforting, enveloping environment that many find soothing. On the other hand, group sports like soccer or basketball could be beneficial for those who need more help with social interaction and communication. These settings offer opportunities to work as part of a team and share space with peers, which are valuable social and emotional learning experiences.

Creating a safe and engaging environment for physical activity is crucial, whether at home or in community settings. At home, designate a specific area for exercise that is free from clutter and potential hazards, ensuring there's enough space for movement without overwhelming sensory stimuli. Utilize this space regularly for physical activities to establish a routine, which can help your child adapt and look forward to this part of their day. In community settings, look for programs or spaces that understand and cater to sensory-sensitive children. These places should offer a structured, predictable schedule for activities, which helps in reducing anxiety about the unknown and allows children to mentally prepare for the session.

Incorporating therapeutic forms of exercise can further enhance the benefits for children with autism. Yoga, for example, is excellent for promoting mindfulness, body awareness, and emotional calm. The structured nature of yoga with its repetitive movements and poses can be particularly appealing to children with ASD, providing them with a sense of security and accomplishment. Adaptive martial arts is another therapeutic activity that not only improves physical fitness but also boosts confidence and self-discipline. Both yoga and adaptive martial arts emphasize self-awareness and controlled movements, which can help in managing impulsivity and agitation, common challenges faced by children with autism.

These physical activities are not merely exercises; they are gateways to improved health, enhanced social skills, and a better quality of life for children with autism. By carefully choosing activities that align with your child's needs, creating a supportive environment, and incorporating therapeutic elements, you can provide your child with valuable tools to help them thrive.

As the chapter on health and autism concludes, we reflect on the profound influence that tailored dietary plans and structured physical activities have on children with ASD. These elements are crucial not just for their physical well-being but for their emotional and social development as well. Looking ahead, the next chapter will explore the legal rights and advocacy necessary to support and protect these needs, ensuring that every child with autism has the opportunity to reach their full potential in all aspects of life.

# MENTAL WELL-BEING

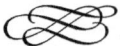

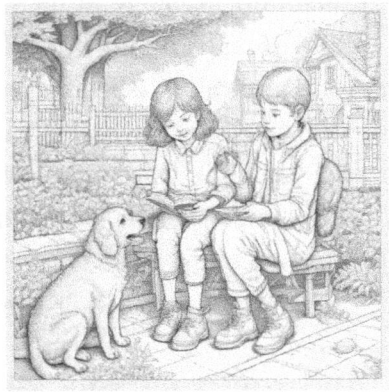

In the quiet moments of reflection, as you watch your child navigate both their world and their inner experiences, you may find yourself pondering deeply about their mental well-being. Understanding and supporting the emotional landscape of a child with Autism Spectrum Disorder (ASD) is as crucial as addressing their physical and educational needs. This chapter is dedicated to unraveling the complexities of mental health challenges that children with autism often encounter, offering you tools and strategies to support them in the most effective and empathetic ways possible.

## 10.1 STRATEGIES FOR SUPPORTING MENTAL HEALTH IN AUTISTIC CHILDREN

### Understanding Mental Health Challenges

The mental health landscape for children with autism can often be intricate and multifaceted, presenting challenges that are distinctively different from their neurotypical peers. Common issues such as anxiety, depression, and emotional dysregulation can manifest uniquely in the context of ASD. For instance, a child with autism may not exhibit sadness or withdrawal symptoms typically associated with depression. Instead, they might display increased irritability, changes in sleep patterns, or a sudden disinterest in activities they previously enjoyed. Anxiety might not come through as worry about future events but could be more immediate and specific, related to changes in routine or sensory overstimulation.

Emotional dysregulation in children with autism often stems from difficulties in identifying and expressing their emotions, leading to overwhelming feelings that might manifest as behavioral outbursts. Unlike neurotypical children who might articulate their feelings of frustration verbally, a child with ASD might communicate these feelings through physical actions, such as aggression or self-injurious behavior. Recognizing these signs as expressions of underlying mental health challenges is crucial in addressing them appropriately and compassionately.

**Building Emotional Awareness and Expression**

Equipping your child with the ability to recognize and express their emotions effectively is a foundational step in supporting their mental health. Techniques such as using emotion cards, which depict various feelings with corresponding facial expressions, can be an excellent tool for younger children. These cards help children with autism connect physical expressions with emotional states, enhancing their ability to recognize these emotions in themselves and others.

Mood journals are another effective tool, especially for older children who can write or draw. Encouraging your child to record their daily emotional experiences can help them process their feelings more explicitly and track patterns over time, which can be particularly useful in understanding what triggers certain emotions. Story-telling, whether through books, movies, or personal stories, can also be a powerful method to explore emotional concepts. These narratives can introduce scenarios that evoke empathy and emotional responses in a controlled, relatable format, allowing children to engage with complex emotions in a safe environment.

**Cognitive Behavioral Techniques**

Cognitive Behavioral Therapy (CBT) techniques can be adapted to help children with autism manage anxiety and stress. Simple methods such as structured breathing exercises help in regulating emotions during moments of distress. For example, teaching your child to take slow, deep breaths can have a calming effect, reducing anxiety and helping them regain control over their reactions.

Mindfulness activities adapted for children with ASD can also be incredibly beneficial. These might include sensory integration-focused practices like listening to calming music or tactile activities like handling stress balls or soft fabric. Such practices not only aid in immediate stress relief but also help in developing a habit of mindfulness over time, enhancing overall emotional regulation.

Positive self-talk is another valuable cognitive technique. Helping your child replace negative thoughts with positive affirmations can boost their self-esteem and reduce feelings of helplessness. For instance, changing a thought from "I can't do this" to "I can try my best" can shift their perspective and improve their approach to challenging situations.

**Establishing a Supportive Routine**

The importance of a consistent daily routine cannot be over-stated when it comes to promoting mental health in children with autism. A routine provides a predictable structure that reduces anxiety and stress, creating a safe and stable environment for your child. This predictability helps in reducing the anxiety that stems from not knowing what to expect, which is often a significant stressor for children with ASD.

Incorporating elements like regular meal times, consistent school routines, and set times for activities such as homework or play can help in establishing this stability. It's also beneficial to include regular slots for relaxation and leisure in the routine, ensuring that your child has ample opportunity to unwind and enjoy their interests. This balance between structured activities and free time is crucial in maintaining an environment that supports both their mental and emotional well-being.

**Interactive Element: Mindfulness Activity Guide**

To integrate mindfulness into your child's routine, here is a simple activity you can start with:

- Mindful Coloring: Choose coloring books with patterns or scenes that your child likes. Set aside a regular time each day for coloring, creating a calm atmosphere with minimal distractions. Encourage your child to focus on the process of coloring, observing the colors and the sensations of the crayon or pencil in their hand. This activity not only promotes mindfulness but also enhances focus and provides a peaceful break from daily routines. (To see where this can lead to, read about Viktor Brevanda in Chapter 16, now an accomplished and up and coming artist, known for his use of vibrant colors)

By understanding the unique ways in which children with autism experience and express their emotions, and by implementing strategies that help them manage these emotions effectively, you are setting a foundation for their long-term mental well-being. This proactive approach not only addresses immediate challenges but also equips your child with skills that will aid them throughout their life, ensuring they have the support and tools they need to navigate their emotions and interactions successfully.

## 10.2 SELF-CARE TIPS FOR PARENTS: MANAGING STRESS AND EMOTIONAL FATIGUE

Navigating the complexities of raising a child with Autism Spectrum Disorder (ASD) is an endeavor that requires immense emotional, physical, and mental commitment. While the focus is often on providing the best possible care for your child, it is equally important to consider your well-being. Understanding how to identify the early signs of stress and emotional fatigue is crucial. Physical indicators might include chronic tiredness, sleep disturbances, or frequent headaches. Emotionally, you may feel over-whelmed, irritable, or detached. Behaviorally, there might be changes such as procrastination on essential tasks, neglect of personal responsibilities, or reduced enjoyment in previously pleasurable activities. Recognizing these signs early can help you take proactive steps towards managing your stress, thereby preserving your health and ensuring you remain an effective support for your child.

The pathway to effective self-care involves integrating practical strategies into your daily routine. Finding time for relaxation is essential. This might mean setting aside specific times each day for activities that help you unwind, such as reading, meditating, or simply sitting quietly for a few minutes. Maintaining social connections is also vital; interacting with friends, family, or support groups can provide emotional relief and a sense of normalcy. Engaging in hobbies or interests that provide a mental break from your caregiving duties can also be incredibly beneficial. These activities not only serve as a distraction but also rejuvenate your mind and spirit, enabling you to return to your responsibilities with renewed energy and perspective.

Setting realistic expectations for both yourself and your child can significantly reduce daily stress. It's important to acknowledge that not every day will be perfect and learning to accept what you realistically can accomplish helps in managing feelings of inadequacy or failure. Alongside this, setting clear boundaries is crucial to prevent overcommitment. Learn to say no or delegate tasks when necessary. Protecting your personal time is not selfish—it is an essential strategy for long-term well-being. This balance allows you to be more present and effective as a parent and caregiver when you are attending to your child's needs.

The importance of professional support cannot be overstated. There might be times when the stress and emotional burden of caregiving become too heavy to manage alone. Seeking help from mental health professionals, such as counselors or therapists, especially those who specialize in caregiving or parental stress, can offer significant relief. These professionals can provide strategies to manage stress effectively and help in processing emotions that may arise from your caregiving role. Additionally, consider support groups specifically designed for parents of children with special needs. These groups provide a platform to share experiences, challenges, and coping strategies, offering both support and validation from others who understand your unique situation.

Managing stress and emotional fatigue is not just about alleviating current symptoms but about implementing a sustainable lifestyle that supports both your well-being and your ability to care for your child. By incorporating these strategies into your life, you ensure that you are looking after your mental and emotional health, which is just as crucial as the physical care you provide for your child. As we turn the page on this chapter, remember that your well-being is integral to the harmony and health of your family. Looking ahead, the next chapter will explore the nuances of transitioning to adulthood for children with ASD, focusing on preparing them for an independent and fulfilling life.

# A NOTE FROM THE AUTHOR

*Autism is not a tragedy. Ignorance is a tragedy.*

— KIM STAGLIANO

My grandson is the reason this book exists. When he was first diagnosed, I'll admit I knew relatively little about ASD, but it was clear to me that finding out everything I could would be my way to forge a deeper connection with him and help him navigate the challenges ahead. Now, at the age of 21, I can truly say he's thriving, and all the work we did with him when he was younger has paid off. He knows himself, and he moves through the world with confidence, accepting his ASD as part of his identity without it being a defining feature.

I want this for your child too. I want it for all children, and the reason I felt compelled to write this book was because I know how much you want it too. You want to understand your child's autism, and you want to connect with them as deeply as you can and equip them with the tools they need to navigate a world that's largely set up for neurotypical people. As a parent to someone with ASD, I know you understand, and I'm sure you want to help other families too – and this is your chance.

**By leaving a review of this book on Amazon, you'll show new readers exactly where they can find all the informa-**

**tion they need to gain a deeper understanding of autism and support their child as fully as they want to.**

As I'm sure you know yourself when your child receives a diagnosis, you're eager to learn all you can, and you start looking for all the help you can find. Your review will help other people to find this easily, spending less time searching and more time soaking up information that they can then put into action.

Thank you so much for your support. It's going to help other parents – and it's going to help their children too.

**Scan the QR code below**

# THE TEENAGE YEARS

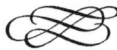

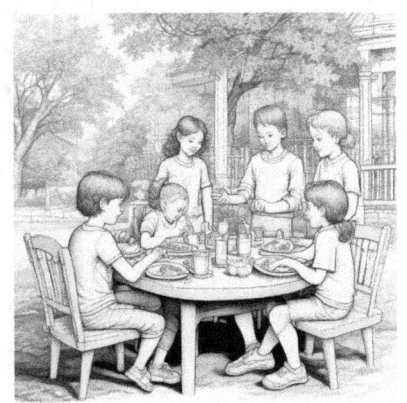

As your child steps into the teenage years, this transformative period brings about a tapestry of changes that are both enriching and challenging. Particularly for a teenager with Autism Spectrum Disorder (ASD), puberty marks a significant milestone that extends beyond mere physical growth; it encompasses a complex interplay of emotional, cognitive, and social developments. This chapter is dedicated to navigating these pivotal years with sensitivity and understanding, ensuring that you, as a parent, are equipped with the knowledge and strategies to support your child through these transformative times.

## 11.1 NAVIGATING PUBERTY AND AUTISM

**Understanding the Impact of Puberty on Autism**

Puberty can often amplify the challenges faced by teenagers with autism, intensifying existing behaviors and introducing new ones. The surge of hormones that marks this stage of development can exacerbate sensory sensitivities and emotional responses, making everyday interactions feel suddenly overwhelming. For some, this can manifest in increased occurrences of meltdowns or withdrawals, as teenagers struggle to cope with the sensory overload. Cognitive shifts during puberty also mean that abstract thinking becomes more pronounced, which can complicate social interactions further. These teenagers might find it increasingly difficult to decode the subtleties of social cues and sarcasm, leading to potential misunderstandings and social isolation.

Moreover, the desire for independence typical of this age can clash with the need for support, creating a tension that both parents and teenagers need to navigate carefully. It's crucial to recognize that while your child is growing up, their unique developmental trajectory may mean they experience and process these changes differently from their neurotypical peers. Adjusting expectations and maintaining open, honest communication during this time becomes key in helping them adjust to the new realities of their evolving world.

## Communication about Bodily Changes

Discussing the physical changes of puberty with your autistic teenager requires clarity, factuality, and sensitivity. It is important to convey the information in a way that aligns with their cognitive processing style. Using visual aids, such as diagrams or illustrated books, can help in explaining the complex concepts of puberty in a more concrete and understandable way. Social stories, which create detailed narratives about various aspects of life, can also be adapted to explain the changes they can expect during puberty.

For instance, creating a social story that walks through the process of getting acne, the reasons behind it, and how to manage it can demystify this common puberty-related change. It is also helpful to prepare your teenager for doctor's visits related to puberty, such as discussions on sexual health, by role-playing these scenarios at home. This preparation can reduce anxiety and make the actual experience more manageable for your teenager.

### Managing Emotional Fluctuations

The emotional rollercoaster that often accompanies puberty can be particularly intense for teenagers with autism. Helping your teenager develop emotional regulation skills is crucial. Techniques such as deep breathing, sensory breaks, and even moderate exercise can be effective tools for managing emotional highs and lows. Structured problem-solving is another critical skill; by helping your teenager learn to identify problems, brainstorm solutions, and evaluate their effectiveness, you empower them to handle emotional challenges with greater autonomy.

Encouraging your teenager to express their emotions through creative outlets like art, music, or writing can also provide them with a safe and constructive way to deal with complex feelings. Additionally, regular check-ins can help you gauge their emotional state and provide timely support. It's important during these discussions to validate their feelings, showing understanding and empathy while guiding them towards effective coping mechanisms.

**Sexual Education and Safety**

Providing comprehensive sexual education that is tailored to the cognitive and emotional level of your autistic teenager is indispensable. This education should encompass not only the basics of human biology but also complex aspects of relationships, consent, and boundaries. Given that teenagers with autism might take longer to understand the nuances of consent and personal boundaries, it's essential that these topics are revisited frequently in a straightforward and explicit manner.

Utilizing resources designed for neurodiverse audiences can enhance this learning process. These resources often use clear, unambiguous language and concrete examples to explain concepts that might otherwise be abstract. Additionally, discussing scenarios involving consent and teaching your teenager how to say "no" or recognize when someone else is saying "no" can provide them with necessary safety skills. This education is not a one-time conversation but a continuous dialogue that adjusts to their growing understanding and experiences.

**Interactive Element: Reflection Section**

To further personalize this learning process and to ensure the information resonates with your family's specific needs, take some time to reflect on the following questions:

- How does my teenager currently handle emotional ups and downs?
- What strategies have we found effective in managing these fluctuations?
- Are there any topics in sexual education that I feel less confident discussing, and how can I seek resources to help?
- How can I create a safe space for my teenager to ask questions and express concerns about puberty?

Reflecting on these questions can help you tailor your approach, ensuring that you are meeting your teenager's unique needs as they navigate the complex journey of adolescence. By maintaining open lines of communication, providing clear and factual information, and supporting them in developing crucial life skills, you can help your teenager face the challenges of puberty with confidence and resilience.

## 11.2 INDEPENDENCE SKILLS FOR TEENAGERS ON THE SPECTRUM

As your child progresses through the teenage years, fostering independence becomes a crucial aspect of their development. The path to independence for a teenager with Autism Spectrum Disorder (ASD) involves a careful assessment of their capabilities across various domains, coupled with tailored instruction in practical life skills and the strategic use of technology to support daily living and decision-making processes.

**Assessing Readiness for Independence**

Determining a teenager's readiness for different levels of independence requires a nuanced understanding of their cognitive, emotional, and practical abilities. Start by observing how your teenager manages tasks they are currently responsible for, such as personal hygiene or homework. Note their reliability in completing these tasks and the quality of outcomes. An effective way to gauge their readiness is to create structured opportunities for them to handle more complex tasks under supervision, gradually increasing the challenge and complexity.

A useful tool in this process is a checklist that addresses various areas of independence:

- Personal Care: Can they manage their hygiene and grooming independently?

- Money Management: Do they understand the concept of money and can handle small amounts responsibly?
- Household Tasks: Are they capable of contributing to household chores?
- Decision-Making: Can they make informed decisions when presented with familiar and safe choices?
- Safety Awareness: Do they understand basic safety rules both inside and outside the home?

This checklist should be revisited periodically to update your assessment and to plan further skill development tailored to their evolving capabilities.

**Teaching Practical Life Skills**

Equipping your teenager with practical life skills is fundamental to independence. Begin by introducing skills that they show readiness for, based on your assessment. For example, if your teenager can follow simple recipes with supervision, you might start with cooking basic meals. Use a step-by-step approach, demonstrating each task, then assisting them as they try, and gradually reducing your involvement as they gain competence.

The key to teaching these skills effectively lies in consistency and patience. Break down tasks into manageable steps and provide clear, concise instructions. Visual aids such as picture guides or step-by-step videos can be very helpful. Regular practice is crucial, and it's beneficial to incorporate these skills into your teenager's daily or weekly routines to reinforce learning.

For money management, begin with understanding the value of different denominations of money and how to handle transactions in safe environments, such as purchasing a snack from a local store. As their confidence grows, introduce concepts like budgeting or saving towards a goal.

**Using Technology to Enhance Independence**

Technology can significantly enhance the independence of autistic teenagers by providing tools that support organization, time management, and daily reminders. Several apps and devices are specifically designed to aid individuals with ASD. For instance, apps that provide visual schedules can help them manage their daily tasks and routines independently. Reminder apps can prompt them about appointments or when to take medication, reducing their reliance on others.

Encourage your teenager to use these technologies under supervision initially, ensuring they understand how to operate them effectively and safely. Discuss the importance of internet safety and personal privacy, setting clear guidelines for responsible use.

**Preparing for Post-School Transitions**

Transitioning from school to higher education or employment is a significant step for any teenager and can be particularly challenging for those with ASD. Begin preparing early by exploring vocational training programs that cater to individuals with special needs, which can provide both job skills and an understanding of workplace dynamics.

For those pursuing higher education, investigate potential accommodations such as extended test time, note-taking services, or quiet study areas. Contact disability services at prospective colleges to discuss how they can support your teenager's needs.

Additionally, familiarize yourself with adult services for individuals with disabilities in your area, including vocational rehabilitation programs and independent living support, to ensure a smooth transition as your teenager moves into adulthood.

By systematically developing these independence skills and leveraging technology, you can significantly enhance your teenager's ability to navigate the adult world with confidence and competence. This not only prepares them for the practical aspects of adulthood but also fosters a sense of self-esteem and accomplishment that is vital for their overall well-being.

As we conclude this exploration into the crucial phase of adolescence, remember that each step your teenager takes towards independence not only prepares them for the practicalities of the adult world but also builds their confidence and self-assurance. In the next chapter, we will shift our focus to navigating the legal landscape, ensuring that you are well-equipped to advocate for your child's rights as they transition into adulthood.

# PREPARING FOR ADULTHOOD

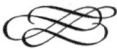

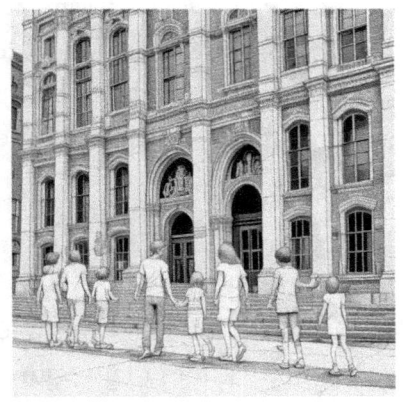

As the dawn of adulthood approaches for your child with Autism Spectrum Disorder (ASD), the landscape of life begins to shift, bringing new challenges and opportunities. This pivotal stage marks a period of significant transition, not just for them but for you as a parent. Navigating this phase effectively requires a blend of preparation, patience, and proactive planning. Here, we delve into the essential life skills that are the bedrock of independent living, offering a roadmap to equip your young adult with the tools they need to thrive in the broader world.

## 12.1 LIFE SKILLS FOR INDEPENDENT LIVING

### Assessing and Developing Essential Daily Living Skills

The journey towards independence starts with mastering daily living skills—those crucial abilities that form the foundation of self-sufficiency. Assessing these skills involves a careful evaluation of your child's current capabilities across various domains: cooking, cleaning, personal hygiene, and money management. Begin this assessment by observing how your child manages these activities under supervision, gradually increasing their responsibility and the complexity of tasks to gauge their competence and confidence.

A systematic approach to teaching these skills can immensely benefit your child. Consider employing task analysis—a method where complex tasks are broken down into smaller, manageable steps. For instance, if teaching cooking, start with simple recipes that require minimal steps and gradually introduce more complex dishes. Utilize visual aids like step-by-step pictorial recipes or instructional videos that can guide your child through the process. Regular practice is crucial and integrating these skills into daily routines can enhance learning, making these tasks familiar and manageable.

**Promoting Self-Care and Personal Responsibility**

Self-care is an integral component of independence. It encompasses various aspects from maintaining personal hygiene to managing stress. Teach your child routines that foster both physical and mental health, such as regular exercise, adequate sleep, and relaxation techniques. Encourage them to take responsibility for their self-care by involving them in the planning and decision-making processes related to their routines.

Promoting personal responsibility also involves managing personal spaces and belongings. Encourage your child to organize their room or manage their laundry, providing support and guidance as needed. This not only teaches them important life skills but also instills a sense of responsibility and pride in managing their environment.

**Safety and Emergency Preparedness**

Safety skills are essential for anyone moving towards independence. Begin by teaching your child how to respond to emergencies—this could include knowing when and how to call emergency services, basic first aid, or evacuation procedures. Use role-playing to walk through various scenarios, helping them understand and memorize the steps involved.

Leverage technology to enhance safety skills. There are numerous mobile apps designed to teach and manage emergency responses, from simple alert systems to more comprehensive apps that guide the user through various emergency situations with visual and audio instructions.

Creating a supportive environment is also crucial. Allow your child to experience natural consequences within safe boundaries. For instance, if they forget their keys, rather than rushing to their rescue, guide them through the process of solving the problem. This approach helps them understand the consequences of their actions and encourages problem-solving skills.

## Social and Community Engagement

As your child steps into adulthood, maintaining and expanding their social networks is vital. Encourage them to engage with community resources such as recreational clubs, volunteer organizations, or interest-based groups. These interactions not only enhance their social skills but also provide a sense of belonging and community.

Discuss the importance of community involvement and social inclusion, guiding them on how to access and navigate these resources. Support them in understanding social norms and expectations, which can be particularly challenging for individuals with ASD. Role-playing can be a useful tool here, helping them practice social interactions in a controlled environment before engaging in real-world settings.

## Interactive Element: Reflection Section

To personalize the strategies discussed and adapt them to your unique situation, consider reflecting on the following questions:

- Which daily living skills does my child handle well, and in which areas do they need more support?
- How can I incorporate the teaching of safety and emergency preparedness into our daily routines?
- What opportunities for social and community engagement exist in our area, and which align with my child's interests and abilities?

Reflecting on these questions can help tailor your approach, ensuring that your child receives the support they need to navigate the challenges of adulthood successfully. By taking proactive steps now, you are paving the way for a future where your child not only manages but thrives independently, equipped with the skills and confidence needed to embrace the adventures of adult life.

## 12.2 EXPLORING VOCATIONAL TRAINING AND EMPLOYMENT OPPORTUNITIES

The transition from adolescence to adulthood is marked by significant milestones, one of the most crucial being the move towards vocational training and employment. For young adults with Autism Spectrum Disorder (ASD), this stage requires careful planning and consideration of their unique strengths, interests, and capabilities. Engaging in a detailed career assessment is the first step towards identifying potential career paths that not only align with their skills but also ignite their passion and interest.

Career assessment should ideally blend both formal tools and informal observations. Formal assessments might include structured interviews, skill assessments, and aptitude tests administered by professionals. These are designed to objectively gauge the abilities and inclinations of your young adult, providing a clear picture of the fields where they might excel. On the other hand, informal observations come from daily interactions and activities. You might notice, for example, that your child shows keen interest in computers, or perhaps they have a knack for organizing things meticulously. These observations are invaluable as they offer real-world insights that formal assessments might overlook.

Once a potential career path is identified, the next step involves exploring appropriate vocational training programs. These programs are tailored to provide the practical skills and real-world experience necessary for job readiness. Programs that incorporate on-the-job training, internships, or apprenticeships are particularly beneficial as they offer hands-on experience, which is crucial for young adults with ASD. These experiences not only refine their skills but also help them adapt to the nuances of workplace environments. When choosing a vocational program, consider the support services they offer, the program's structure, and how it aligns with your child's learning style and needs.

Navigating the job market can be a daunting task for any young adult, more so for someone with ASD. Practical advice on job searching, crafting a tailored resume, and preparing for interviews can greatly ease this process. Encourage your child to create a resume that highlights their strengths and any practical experiences, like internships or volunteer work, which are relevant to the job they are seeking. Interview preparation should include role-playing exercises to simulate potential interview scenarios. This practice can build confidence and reduce anxiety about the actual interviews. Thankfully we are entering an era where corporations are starting to understand and appreciate some of the strengths of neurodivergence. The Wall Street Journal published an excellent article on June 9, 2024 titled "Jobs for the Autistic Grow beyond Tech". If you have a child at that stage of life, you will be well advised and encouraged to read or listen to the article. ( Unfortunately because the Wall Street Journal is subscription based, we are not able to generate a QR code for you to open and read the article)

Disclosing autism to potential employers is a personal decision and should be handled with care. If your young adult chooses to disclose, it should be done strategically to advocate for any necessary accommodations that would enable them to perform their best work. These accommodations might include a quiet workspace, detailed written instructions for tasks, or flexible scheduling. Educating potential employers about ASD can also help in fostering a supportive and inclusive work environment.

In the workplace, understanding the culture and building relationships with coworkers are as critical as the job skills themselves. Guidance in navigating these social dynamics is key to workplace success. Teach your young adult about the importance of communication, teamwork, and the unwritten norms that often govern workplace interactions. Advocating for themselves in terms of necessary accommodations or support is also a skill that they will need to develop. This advocacy is crucial not only for their comfort and productivity but also for their career advancement over time.

As your young adult steps into the world of vocational training and employment, the skills and strategies discussed here will serve as a solid foundation for their journey. This preparation not only sets the stage for personal and professional growth but also contributes to a broader sense of fulfillment and independence. Looking ahead, the next chapter will focus on the legal rights and advocacy, crucial elements that ensure these young adults can navigate their paths with the support and recognition they deserve, enhancing their ability to succeed in an ever-evolving society.

# LEGAL RIGHTS AND ADVOCACY

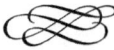

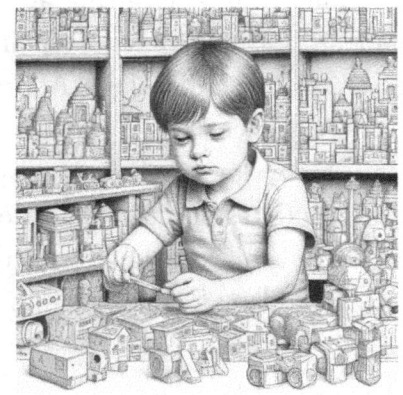

Navigating the complexities of the legal landscape can often feel like trying to find a clear path through a dense forest. For parents of children with Autism Spectrum Disorder (ASD), understanding and advocating for your child's legal rights is not just a necessity—it's an empowerment tool that unlocks doors to essential services and protections. This chapter is dedicated to demystifying the legal rights that safeguard individuals with autism across various settings, ensuring you are well-equipped to advocate effectively for your child's needs and entitlements.

## 13.1 UNDERSTANDING LEGAL RIGHTS IN DIFFERENT SETTINGS

**Rights in Educational Settings**

Education is not just a fundamental right; it's a critical runway to personal growth and development. For children with ASD, the Individuals with Disabilities Education Act (IDEA) and Section 504 of the Rehabilitation Act serve as the bedrock of educational rights, ensuring access to tailored educational opportunities. IDEA mandates that all children with disabilities are entitled to a Free Appropriate Public Education (FAPE) that meets their unique needs. Under IDEA, schools must develop an Individualized Education Program (IEP) that outlines specific educational goals and the services needed to achieve them, ensuring a structured plan that accommodates the child's educational requirements.

Section 504, on the other hand, broadens this approach by prohibiting discrimination based on disability in any program receiving federal financial assistance. This means that any public school or educational program must provide accommodations and modifications to ensure that children with disabilities have educational opportunities comparable to those provided to non-disabled students. These accommodations might include anything from extra time on tests to specialized educational aids. Understanding these laws helps you ensure that your child does not miss out on educational benefits due to oversight or lack of resources.

## Healthcare Rights

When it comes to healthcare, the Americans with Disabilities Act (ADA) ensures that individuals with autism have the right to accessible medical care. This encompasses not only physical access to medical facilities but also accommodations that might be necessary during medical appointments, such as the presence of a caregiver or communication aids. Furthermore, the ADA mandates reasonable modifications in policies, practices, and procedures to ensure that individuals with disabilities receive equal access to health services.

Navigating insurance and healthcare laws is another critical aspect that can significantly impact treatment options. It's essential to understand your insurance policy's provisions regarding therapies and interventions commonly used in autism care, such as behavioral therapy or occupational therapy. Some states have specific mandates that require insurance companies to cover autism services, and knowing these provisions can help in advocating for necessary treatments. Also, be aware of the appeal processes available if coverage is initially denied. This knowledge ensures that you are better prepared to navigate the complexities of insurance and secure the treatments your child needs.

## Employment Rights

As children with ASD transition into adulthood, the ADA continues to protect their rights in the workplace. This includes the right to reasonable accommodations that enable an employee with a disability to perform their job duties effectively. Accommodations can vary widely, from modified work schedules and the provision of specialized equipment to adjustments in training materials or procedures. It's important for young adults with autism and their families to understand that employers have an obligation under the ADA to provide accommodations unless doing so would cause undue hardship to the business.

In addition to accommodations, the ADA protects individuals with disabilities from discrimination in hiring, promotions, job assignments, termination, and other aspects of employment. If discrimination is suspected, it can be reported to the Equal Employment Opportunity Commission (EEOC), which enforces these regulations. Being informed about these rights and knowing how to address and report violations can empower your young adult to seek fair treatment in their professional endeavors.

**Community and Public Life**

The right to access public spaces and services is fundamental to ensuring that individuals with autism can participate fully in community life. This includes accessibility to public transportation, the right to vote, and access to public areas such as parks and libraries. The ADA mandates that public facilities must be accessible to individuals with disabilities, and this extends to ensuring that community programs and services are inclusive and accommodate the needs of those with autism.

For example, modifications might be necessary at polling stations to assist individuals with autism during voting, such as providing a quiet environment or allowing a caregiver to assist in the voting process. Understanding these rights helps ensure that your child or young adult can engage with and contribute to their community without facing unnecessary barriers.

**Interactive Element: Checklist for Navigating Legal Rights**

To assist you in navigating and advocating for these rights, consider using the following checklist:

**Educational Rights:**

- Review your child's IEP annually to ensure it meets their evolving educational needs.
- Familiarize yourself with both IDEA and Section 504 to understand the scope of educational accommodations and services available.

**Healthcare Rights:**

- Ensure that your healthcare providers are aware of the ADA requirements related to accessible medical care.
- Review your insurance coverage annually to understand what autism-related treatments and therapies are covered.

**Employment Rights:**

- Educate your young adult about their rights under the ADA regarding employment and reasonable accommodations.
- Familiarize yourself with the process of filing a complaint with the EEOC in case of suspected discrimination.

**Community Access:**

- Engage with local community centers to discuss how they can be more inclusive of individuals with autism.
- Ensure that your local polling station is aware of and compliant with ADA regulations during elections.

This checklist serves as a practical tool to help you ensure that your child or young adult's rights are not only understood but actively upheld. As you navigate through these legal landscapes, remain proactive and informed, empowering yourself to act confidently and effectively on behalf of your child's interests and rights.

## 13.2 EFFECTIVE ADVOCACY TECHNIQUES FOR PARENTS

The role of an advocate is one you naturally assume as a parent of a child with Autism Spectrum Disorder (ASD). Equipping yourself with a robust understanding of autism-related laws and rights is not just beneficial—it's necessary for ensuring that your child receives the appropriate support and resources they are entitled to. This foundational knowledge can be significantly bolstered by engaging with advocacy groups, attending educational workshops, and sometimes consulting with legal experts who specialize in disability rights. These resources serve as a lifeline, providing updates on legislative changes, insights into advocacy strategies, and platforms for networking with other parents and professionals. They transform the complex legal landscape into navigable terrain, ensuring you are always a step ahead in advocating for your child's needs.

Documentation is another pillar of effective advocacy. Keeping meticulous records of everything from educational plans and medical treatments to interactions with professionals is crucial. These documents are invaluable in legal and advocacy contexts, serving as evidence to support your claims or requests. For instance, detailed records of your child's Individualized Education Program (IEP) meetings and adjustments can be crucial during discussions about educational placements or services. Similarly, keeping a log of medical appointments, treatments, and recommendations can aid in securing insurance coverage or in disputes regarding your child's health care. Start by maintaining organized files, both digital and physical, and make it a habit to document all pertinent communications and decisions. This not only prepares you for potential challenges but also ensures you have a historical account of your child's journey that can inform future decisions.

Effective communication and negotiation skills are indispensable tools in your advocacy arsenal. When dealing with institutions like schools, healthcare providers, or employers, clarity and assertiveness in communication can make a significant difference. Prepare for meetings by outlining your objectives and concerns clearly and consider potential questions or objections. Practice active listening, which not only aids in understanding others' perspectives but also in formulating reasoned responses. When negotiating accommodations or services, be specific about what is needed and why, and be prepared to offer alternatives that might still meet these needs. If issues escalate, know how to assert your rights firmly and respectfully, and understand the formal grievance procedures available.

Leveraging community and legal resources is often necessary, especially when confronting violations of rights or navigating complex situations that require expert intervention. Local and online support groups can be invaluable, offering advice based on collective experiences and sometimes providing connections to recommended legal counsel specialized in disability rights. Nonprofit organizations often conduct workshops and provide resources that can enhance your understanding and advocacy efforts. In situations where legal action might be necessary, such as discrimination cases or disputes over service provision, seeking legal counsel early can provide guidance on your options and the best course of action.

### Resource List: Advocacy Support

- Autism Advocacy Network: Offers resources for understanding legal rights and provides advocacy training.

- Family Support Workshops: Local workshops that focus on teaching negotiation skills and rights awareness.
- Online Parent Forums: Platforms where experiences and strategies are shared, offering community support and advice.

Learning to navigate these advocacy paths effectively ensures that you not only fight for your child's rights but also empower them to thrive in a society that recognizes and respects their needs. As this chapter closes, remember that every step you take builds a bridge towards a more inclusive world for your child. Looking forward, the next chapter will explore community engagement and inclusion, vital elements that enrich your child's social interactions and broaden their horizons.

# COMMUNITY AND SUPPORT

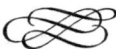

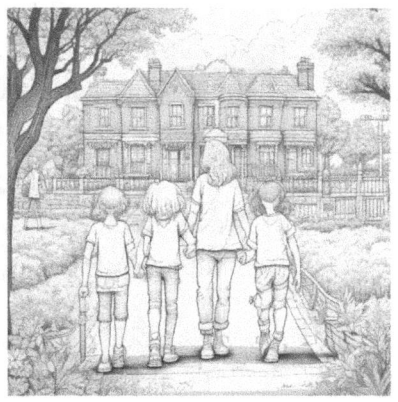

As you navigate the complexities and joys of raising a child with Autism Spectrum Disorder (ASD), discovering and integrating into supportive communities can be transformative. Just as a tree draws strength from its roots, so too can families thrive with the support of a robust network. This chapter delves deep into the essence of finding, joining, and even creating support networks that resonate with the specific needs of families touched by autism. Here, you will learn not just to find these communities but to engage with them in ways that enrich both your family's life and those of others in the network.

## 14.1 FINDING AND BUILDING SUPPORT NETWORKS

**Identifying Relevant Support Networks**

Embarking on the quest to find the right support network involves more than a simple search; it requires a nuanced understanding of your family's specific needs and the goals you wish to achieve through this community. Support networks for families affected by autism vary widely, ranging from formal organizations offering resources and advocacy to informal online groups that provide moral and emotional support. When selecting a network, consider the focus of the group—whether it's on early childhood, teenage years, or adulthood—as this alignment with your child's age can provide more targeted support and relevant sharing of experiences.

Additionally, evaluate the types of activities and resources offered by the network. Some groups might focus on educational workshops and seminars that can help you better understand ASD and the latest interventions. Others might emphasize social gatherings or playgroups, which can be invaluable for your child's social development and your own respite and connection with other parents. The structure of the group is also crucial; a well-organized network with a clear mission and active leadership can offer more substantial support and more reliable engagement than a less formal group.

## Benefits of Joining Support Networks

The benefits of embedding yourself and your child within a support network extend far beyond the immediate sharing of information and resources. Emotionally, these networks provide a sense of belonging and understanding that is often missing in broader social contexts where ASD might be misunderstood. They offer a space where your experiences are validated by others who are on similar paths, providing comfort and reducing the isolation that can sometimes accompany the parenting journey of a child with ASD.

For your child, being part of a network that includes opportunities for interaction with peers can foster important social skills and friendships. These social settings allow them to engage in a safe and understanding environment where their unique traits are accepted and celebrated. Moreover, your active participation in these networks can model social engagement and advocacy, teaching your child valuable interpersonal and self-advocacy skills that are essential throughout life.

## Steps to Engage with Support Networks

Engaging effectively with a support network involves more than just attendance; it requires active participation. Start by attending meetings regularly to understand the group's dynamics and the needs of its members. Participate in discussions, share your experiences, and offer your insights, which can help others and strengthen the network. Volunteering for activities or organizational roles within the network can also enhance your involvement and give you a deeper sense of contribution and belonging.

Moreover, consider the ways you can bring value to the group based on your skills and experiences. Whether it's organizing events, offering to speak on topics you are knowledgeable about, or simply providing a listening ear to new members, your active contribution can significantly enhance the network's support capacity.

## Creating Your Own Support Network

In regions or situations where existing networks are sparse or do not meet your family's needs, establishing a local support group might be the best course of action. Begin by identifying other families and individuals who might be interested in joining. Venues such as local community centers, libraries, or schools often provide space for community groups at little or no cost.

Promotion is key to gathering members; utilize social media, community bulletin boards, and connections through therapists or doctors specialized in ASD. Organize regular meetings or events, and decide on the group's structure and goals based on the members' inputs. Being the founder of a support network can be a rewarding experience that not only fills a gap in your community but also positions you as a leader within the local ASD support landscape.

**Interactive Element: Reflection Section**

To help integrate the ideas presented, reflect on the following:

- What are the top three qualities I am looking for in a support network?
- How can I contribute to a support network in a way that utilizes my strengths and experiences?
- What steps can I take this month to either join a new support network or enhance my involvement in an existing one?

Engaging with supportive communities offers a pathway not just to resources and information, but to emotional support, friendship, and mutual growth. These networks can become your family's extended family, providing support and understanding as you navigate the unique challenges and joys of raising a child with ASD.

## 14.2 THE POWER OF COMMUNITY: ENGAGING WITH LOCAL AND ONLINE GROUPS

Navigating the landscape of Autism Spectrum Disorder (ASD) with your child can often feel like charting unknown territories. However, embedding yourself and your child within local and online communities can transform this path, turning it into a well-trodden road supported by collective wisdom and shared experiences. These communities offer a wealth of resources that can significantly enhance your child's development and your family's well-being.

## Leveraging Local Community Resources

Local community resources such as libraries, community centers, and educational institutions are treasure troves of activities and programs that can be incredibly beneficial for children with autism. These places often host events, workshops, and social gatherings that provide not only learning opportunities but also social interaction in a structured and supportive environment. For instance, many libraries offer sensory-friendly reading hours designed specifically for children with ASD, providing a quieter, more accommodating setting to enjoy books.

Advocating for the inclusion of autism-friendly events and services involves a proactive approach. Start by connecting with the coordinators or managers of these institutions. Present them with clear, concise information about ASD and the specific needs of children affected by it. Highlight the benefits not only for your child but for the community at large—increased inclusivity, awareness, and understanding. Many organizations are open to hosting such events but may lack the knowledge or push to initiate them. Your advocacy can be the catalyst for change, leading to regular events that cater to sensory sensitivities, communication differences, and other ASD-related needs.

Moreover, consider collaborating with these institutions to organize workshops or talks about ASD. These events can serve dual purposes: educating the public about autism and providing parents like yourself a platform to share experiences, tips, and strategies. Such initiatives not only enrich the community's understanding but also weave your child's experiences into the fabric of local society, fostering acceptance and inclusion.

## Engaging with Online Communities

The digital age offers an expansive universe of online communities that bring together individuals from diverse backgrounds, including parents of children with autism. These virtual platforms—ranging from forums and social media groups to blogs focused on ASD—can provide support, advice, and a sense of belonging. They allow you to connect with families navigating similar challenges, share experiences, and exchange resources that can be invaluable in your day-to-day life.

However, the vastness of the internet also comes with challenges. It's crucial to identify and engage with online communities that are reputable and constructive. Look for groups that are well-moderated, with clear guidelines on interaction and content sharing. These communities should offer a positive atmosphere where information is shared responsibly and supportively. Participate actively but cautiously—share your experiences and learn from others, but also protect your and your child's privacy by not divulging sensitive personal information.

Engaging productively also means contributing to the positivity and resourcefulness of the group. Share useful articles, upcoming events, or personal anecdotes that offer encouragement and insight. The strength of online communities often lies in the collective support and diverse perspectives they harness.

## Building Relationships within the Community

Whether local or online, the relationships you forge within these communities can be a source of ongoing support and growth. Building and maintaining these relationships requires mutual respect, shared experiences, and a commitment to support each other. Actively participate in community activities, offer your help to new members, and be a consistent presence that others can rely on. In return, you'll find that the community becomes a reliable support system for you too, offering advice and empathy on tough days and celebrating with you on the good ones.

## Community Advocacy

Taking on an advocacy role within your community can amplify the impact of your efforts, pushing for broader acceptance and better resources for individuals with autism. Work with local businesses, schools, and policymakers to raise awareness about ASD. This might involve organizing awareness campaigns, participating in school board meetings, or collaborating with local health services to improve their ASD accommodations.

Your advocacy not only influences public perceptions but also policy decisions that can lead to greater resources and support for the autism community. By championing these causes, you help pave the way for a society that not only understands autism but actively supports and includes individuals affected by it.

As this chapter wraps up, remember that the strength of community lies not just in the resources it offers but in the connections it fosters—connections that can support, educate, and empower both you and your child as you navigate ASD. These communities provide a framework within which you can advocate for change, share your journey, and find a collective voice that champions inclusion and understanding.

Looking ahead, the next chapter will delve into cultural perspectives on autism, exploring how different cultures understand and manage ASD and how these perspectives can influence treatment and acceptance. This exploration will not only broaden your understanding of how autism is viewed globally but also enhance your approach to managing and supporting your child's unique needs.

# CULTURAL PERSPECTIVES ON AUTISM

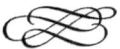

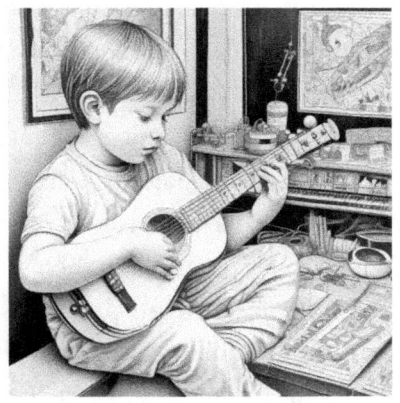

As we navigate the multifaceted realm of Autism Spectrum Disorder (ASD), we encounter a tapestry woven with diverse cultural threads, each adding its unique hue and texture to our understanding of autism. The way autism is perceived, diagnosed, and treated can vary dramatically across different cultures, influenced by a myriad of factors ranging from societal norms to available resources. This chapter delves into the cultural landscapes that shape the autism experience worldwide, exploring the challenges and opportunities that arise when diverse cultural perspectives intersect with the scientific and medical understanding of autism.

## 15.1 AUTISM IN DIVERSE CULTURES: UNDERSTANDING AND CHALLENGES

### Variability in Autism Recognition and Diagnosis

Autism, a condition known for its wide spectrum of manifestations, is viewed through various lenses in different parts of the world. In many Western countries, significant advances in autism research and a relatively high level of awareness have led to earlier diagnoses and interventions. However, this is not a universal reality. In some regions of Asia, Africa, and South America, cultural beliefs and a lack of resources can lead to underdiagnosis or misdiagnosis of autism. For instance, in rural areas of India, traditional beliefs about child development and behavior might lead families and even some healthcare providers to view early signs of autism as merely quirks or phases that a child will outgrow. Similarly, in parts of Africa, limited access to trained professionals and diagnostic tools means that autism might not be recognized, leaving children without the support and interventions that are crucial in their early years.

The contrast in diagnostic practices can be stark when comparing regions with robust healthcare systems to those where healthcare is less accessible. For example, in Scandinavian countries, where healthcare systems are highly developed, autism diagnosis tends to be more consistent and aligned with international standards. Conversely, in some parts of Eastern Europe and Central Asia, inconsistencies in diagnostic criteria and a lack of specialized training can result in a fragmented picture of autism prevalence and awareness.

## Cultural Stigmas and Their Impact on Families

Cultural stigmas surrounding mental health and disabilities can profoundly impact families dealing with autism. In many cultures, there is a significant stigma attached to mental health disorders, which can extend to autism. This stigma often leads to social isolation for both the individual and their family. In Middle Eastern societies, for instance, family honor and social reputation are highly valued, and having a family member diagnosed with a neurological condition like autism can be seen as a mark of shame. This perception can deter families from seeking diagnosis and support, leading to a lack of treatment and increased familial stress.

Families in these situations often face a dual challenge: managing the needs of a child with autism and navigating the cultural expectations and judgments of their community. The fear of ostracism not only affects the willingness to seek diagnosis but also influences how families interact within their community, often choosing to hide their child's condition to avoid negative reactions.

## Traditional vs. Western Approaches to Treatment

The approach to autism treatment varies widely across cultures, influenced by differing beliefs about health and wellness. In Western countries, treatments such as behavioral therapies and speech therapy are commonly prescribed and are supported by a wealth of scientific research. However, in non-Western cultures, traditional and holistic approaches often prevail. For example, in some parts of China, acupuncture and herbal medicine are commonly used to treat symptoms associated with autism. These methods are deeply rooted in the traditional Chinese belief system about the balance of bodily energies and are often preferred over more conventional Western medical treatments.

Community-based solutions also play a significant role in regions where formal healthcare infrastructure is lacking or where there is a strong sense of community involvement in caregiving. In parts of Africa, for instance, the extended family and community often take on significant roles in the care and support of individuals with autism, sometimes more so than professional healthcare providers. This communal approach can offer a strong support network but may also lack access to specialized therapies that could benefit the individual's development.

**Challenges in Global Advocacy**

Advocating for autism awareness and acceptance presents unique challenges on a global scale. Efforts to raise awareness and promote inclusivity must navigate a complex landscape of cultural norms, economic constraints, and varying levels of government support. Organizations working in this field often find that strategies that are effective in one country may not be suitable in another. For example, advocacy approaches that work well in the United States, such as media campaigns and celebrity endorsements, may not resonate in countries with different media landscapes or cultural values.

Bridging these cultural divides requires a nuanced understanding of each region's specific needs and sensitivities. Collaborative efforts between local and international organizations can be effective, as they combine local knowledge with global resources. For instance, partnerships between local schools and international NGOs can help bring advanced training and resources to teachers in under-resourced areas, improving the quality of education and support available to children with autism.

These efforts are crucial in paving the way toward a more inclusive world where individuals with autism are recognized and valued, regardless of where they live. As we continue to explore and understand the diverse cultural perspectives on autism, we broaden our capacity to advocate for effective, culturally appropriate solutions that can transform lives across the globe.

## 15.2 INCORPORATING CULTURAL SENSITIVITY INTO AUTISM CARE

Navigating the complexities of autism care requires not only an understanding of the condition itself but also an appreciation of the cultural contexts in which individuals with autism and their families live. Recognizing and respecting cultural differences in communication styles and practices is essential, as these differences can significantly influence how autism symptoms are perceived and treated. Cultural competence in healthcare and educational settings isn't just a beneficial skill—it's a necessity. It allows professionals to connect with and effectively support diverse families, ensuring that interventions are both respectful and effective.

For instance, in some cultures, direct communication is considered rude, and indirect methods are preferred. This can affect how symptoms are reported and discussed in clinical or educational settings. A professional skilled in cultural competence will recognize these nuances and adapt their approach, perhaps by using more open-ended questions or allowing more time for the family to express their concerns without direct questioning. This sensitivity not only facilitates better communication but also builds trust, which is crucial for effective therapy and education.

Moreover, the development of interventions and supports must take cultural contexts into account to ensure they are relevant and sensitive to the needs of the community. This might involve adapting educational materials to include culturally familiar examples or ensuring that therapy practices respect familial roles and expectations. For example, in a community where family hierarchy is significant, interventions might need to involve key family members and respect their input more than might be typical in Western settings. These adaptations help ensure that interventions are not only technically effective but also culturally resonant, increasing their likelihood of success.

Engaging multicultural families effectively in the care and education of their children with autism also involves overcoming potential language barriers and respecting familial and cultural values. Strategies such as employing interpreters or bilingual professionals can facilitate clearer communication, ensuring that all family members understand and are engaged in the treatment process. It's also crucial to be aware of cultural norms that might influence interactions, such as who in the family makes decisions about a child's care or how mental health issues are perceived. Professionals need to approach these situations with sensitivity and flexibility, adapting their methods to align with family dynamics and expectations.

Training professionals in cultural competency is therefore an integral part of enhancing autism care in diverse settings. Programs and strategies that have been successful often include comprehensive training on cultural awareness, specific communication strategies, and case studies that highlight effective cross-cultural interventions. These programs not only prepare professionals to work more effectively with diverse populations but also help them understand the broader social and cultural factors that affect families living with autism.

Incorporating these elements of cultural sensitivity ensures that all families, regardless of their cultural background, receive supportive, respectful, and effective care. This approach not only improves outcomes for individuals with autism but also enriches the caregiving community by fostering an environment of inclusivity and understanding.

As we conclude this exploration of cultural sensitivity in autism care, we reflect on the importance of understanding and embracing the diverse cultural landscapes that shape the experiences of individuals with autism and their families. This chapter underscores the necessity of cultural competence in providing effective, respectful, and inclusive care and education for all. As we move forward, the insights gained here will continue to inform our approaches and interactions, ensuring that every individual with autism is supported in a manner that honors their cultural identity and personal needs.

# STORIES OF HOPE AND SUCCESS

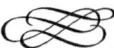

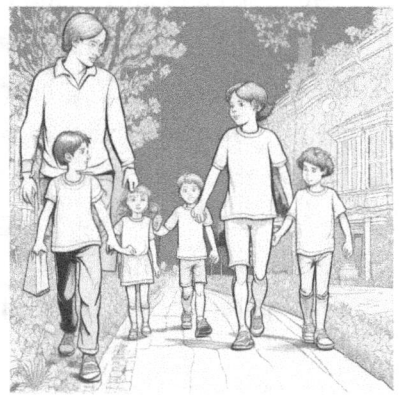

In the vast universe of Autism Spectrum Disorder, the stars that shine the brightest are often those of individuals who have turned their unique challenges into avenues of success. This chapter is a celebration of such stars—individuals with autism who have not only faced their challenges head-on but have also carved paths of achievement in academics, arts, sports, and entrepreneurship. These stories are not just narratives of personal victories; they are beacons of inspiration and powerful testimonials to the diverse potential within the autism community.

## 16.1 PERSONAL TRIUMPHS: STORIES OF SUCCESS AND RESILIENCE

### Highlighting Diverse Achievements

While our goal in this book is to highlight the diversity of characteristics on the ASD spectrum, we would be remiss not to start with a brief history of one of the world's most successful entrepreneurs of our current age, Elon Musk. The second individual who we highlight is quite young and an incredibly talented artist, Viktor Bevanda. His skills are quite different from Elon's and yet therein lies the awesomeness of this neurodiversity. Both individuals are autistic and yet are as diverse and distinct as can be from each other. The third individual we highlight is John Elder Robison whose talents as a teenager were as diverse as Musk and Bevanda, and yet all three fall into the spectrum we call Autism Spectrum Disorder.

Our other contributors shall remain nameless solely to protect their identity. There are many folks out there who wish to stay out of the public limelight, and we must respect that.

### *Elon Musk*

Elon Musk, the man who would become one of the most innovative and influential entrepreneurs of the 21st century, was born on June 28, 1971, in Pretoria, South Africa. From a young age, it was clear that Elon was different from other children. He exhibited a profound curiosity and a unique way of perceiving the world around him, characteristics that would later be identified as traits of Asperger's syndrome.

Growing up, Elon's mind was constantly buzzing with ideas and questions. While other children played outside, Elon would immerse himself in books, absorbing knowledge like a sponge. By the age of ten, he had developed a deep interest in computing and technology. His parents, Maye and Errol Musk, were both supportive but often found it challenging to understand their son's intense focus and his difficulty with social interactions.

School was a difficult environment for Elon. He was often bullied and ostracized by his peers for being different. His lack of social skills and his tendency to engage in long, detailed monologues about his interests made it hard for him to make friends. These challenges, however, did not deter Elon. Instead, he found solace in his passions. At the age of twelve, he taught himself computer programming and created a video game called Blastar, which he sold for $500.

Elon's teenage years were marked by a move to Canada, where he enrolled at Queen's University. This change in environment was both a challenge and an opportunity. It was difficult for Elon to adapt to a new country and culture, but it also allowed him to start fresh. At Queen's University, Elon met Justine Wilson, his first wife, and began to develop a social circle that appreciated his unique intellect and vision.

After two years at Queen's, Elon transferred to the University of Pennsylvania, where he earned degrees in both physics and economics. His time at university was characterized by a relentless pursuit of knowledge. Elon's Asperger's syndrome gave him an extraordinary ability to focus intensely on subjects that interested him, allowing him to excel academically.

Following his graduation, Elon moved to California to pursue a PhD at Stanford University. However, he quickly realized that his true calling was in entrepreneurship, not academia. He dropped out of Stanford after just two days to start his first company, Zip2, a city guide software for news-papers. This was the beginning of a series of ventures that would define his career.

Elon's Asperger's syndrome played a crucial role in his approach to business and innovation. His ability to hyper-focus allowed him to delve deeply into complex subjects and solve problems that others might have deemed insurmount-able. This trait was particularly evident in his work with SpaceX and Tesla.

In 2002, Elon founded SpaceX with the goal of reducing space transportation costs and making space exploration more accessible. His vision was ambitious, but his singular focus and attention to detail enabled him to overcome the many obstacles that stood in his way. For example, when SpaceX's first three rockets failed to reach orbit, many critics predicted the company's demise. However, Elon's unyielding determination and belief in his vision drove him to continue. In 2008, SpaceX successfully launched Falcon 1 into orbit, marking a significant milestone in private spaceflight.

Similarly, Elon's work with Tesla revolutionized the auto-motive industry. He saw the potential for electric vehicles to reduce dependency on fossil fuels and combat climate change. Despite widespread skepticism and significant financial challenges, Elon's perseverance paid off. Under his leadership, Tesla developed groundbreaking technologies and produced electric cars that were both high-performing and commercially successful. Today, Tesla is a leading player in the automotive industry, pushing the boundaries of innovation and sustainability.

Elon's Asperger's syndrome also influenced his leadership style. He was known for his direct communication and high expectations, which sometimes led to friction with employees and colleagues. However, his clear vision and unwavering commitment to his goals inspired many to strive for excellence. Elon's ability to think differently and challenge conventional wisdom was a driving force behind his companies' success.

In addition to SpaceX and Tesla, Elon founded or co-founded several other ventures, including SolarCity, Neuralink, and The Boring Company. Each of these companies reflected his desire to solve complex global problems through innovative technology. Whether it was developing sustainable energy solutions, advancing brain-computer interfaces, or addressing urban transportation issues, Elon's unique perspective and relentless drive were central to his approach.

Despite his many successes, Elon's journey was not without personal challenges. His intense focus on work often came at the expense of his personal life, leading to strained relationships and significant stress. Managing the demands of multiple high-stakes ventures required a level of dedication and resilience that few could sustain. However, Elon's

Asperger's syndrome, which had been a source of difficulty in his youth, became a source of strength in his professional life, enabling him to maintain his vision and achieve his goals.

Elon Musk's story is a testament to the power of embracing one's unique qualities and turning challenges into strengths. His journey from a socially isolated child in South Africa to a world-renowned entrepreneur and innovator is a remarkable example of how Asperger's syndrome, with its accompanying traits of intense focus and unconventional thinking, can be a powerful asset. Elon's life and career illustrate that what sets us apart can also be what drives us to achieve greatness. His legacy continues to inspire countless individuals to pursue their passions, think differently, and strive to make a positive impact on the world.

### Viktor Bevanda

Viktor Bevanda is a remarkable young artist whose journey is as unique as the masterpieces he creates. Born with autism, Viktor's story is a testament to how neurodiversity can be a source of incredible talent and creativity. His art skills, which have captivated many, are not merely a coincidence but are deeply intertwined with his autism.

### Early Life and Diagnosis

Viktor was diagnosed with autism at the age of three. His parents, initially overwhelmed by the diagnosis, soon realized that their son viewed the world through a different lens. Unlike neurotypical children, Viktor had a heightened sensitivity to his surroundings. Sounds, colors, and textures that others might overlook became focal points for him. This heightened perception played a crucial role in the development of his art.

## The Emergence of Talent

From a young age, Viktor displayed an extraordinary ability to focus. While other children were engaged in typical play activities, Viktor found solace and joy in drawing. His parents noticed that he would spend hours meticulously working on his sketches, often losing track of time. This deep concentration is a common trait among many autistic individuals, allowing them to excel in their areas of interest.

Viktor's autism endowed him with a unique way of seeing the world. He could observe minute details that others might miss. This keen observation translated into his art, where every piece is filled with intricate patterns and vibrant colors. His sensory sensitivity allowed him to perceive and replicate the nuances of light, shadow, and texture with remarkable accuracy.

## Art as a Communication Tool

For Viktor, art became more than just a hobby; it was a vital means of communication. Autism often affects verbal communication skills, and Viktor was no exception. He struggled with expressing his thoughts and emotions through words, which led to frustration and isolation. However, through his art, he found a voice. Each drawing and painting became a story, a way for Viktor to share his inner world with those around him.

His parents encouraged his artistic pursuits, providing him with various mediums to explore. From pencils and markers to paints and digital tools, Viktor experimented with different techniques, each time discovering new ways to express himself. This support from his family was crucial in nurturing his talent and building his confidence.

## The Influence of Autism on Art Style

Viktor's art style is profoundly influenced by his autism. Many of his works feature repetitive patterns and symmetrical designs, which are reflective of the repetitive behaviors and preference for order often seen in autistic individuals. These patterns are not just visually appealing but also provide Viktor with a sense of calm and predictability.

His use of color is another aspect where his autism shines through. Viktor has an exceptional ability to blend and contrast colors, creating pieces that are both striking and harmonious. His sensory sensitivity allows him to experiment with bold color choices that evoke strong emotional responses from viewers.

Moreover, Viktor's unique way of processing information means that he often sees the bigger picture differently. While others might focus on the main subject of a scene, Viktor captures the entire environment with equal importance. This holistic approach results in artworks that are rich in detail and depth, drawing viewers into a world seen through Viktor's eyes.

## Recognition and Impact

As Viktor's talent grew, so did the recognition of his work. Local art shows and exhibitions soon featured his pieces, and his name began to spread within the art community. His story became an inspiration for many, highlighting the incredible potential within individuals with autism. Schools and organizations started inviting him to speak and share his experiences, using his art to raise awareness about autism and the importance of embracing neurodiversity.

Viktor's art also had a profound impact on his personal development. The recognition and appreciation he received boosted his self-esteem and encouraged him to continue exploring his creative abilities. Through art, he found a sense of purpose and a way to connect with others, breaking through the barriers that autism often presents.

**The Role of Support Systems**

Viktor's journey would not have been possible without the unwavering support of his family, teachers, and therapists. They recognized his potential early on and provided the resources and encouragement he needed to thrive. His parents, in particular, played a crucial role in fostering his talent, ensuring that he had access to art supplies and opportunities to showcase his work.

His teachers adapted their methods to suit his learning style, allowing him to incorporate art into his studies and use it as a tool for learning and expression. Therapists worked with him to improve his communication skills and manage the challenges that came with autism, all while encouraging his artistic endeavors.

**Looking to the Future**

Today, Viktor Bevanda continues to create and inspire. His artwork is not just a reflection of his talent but also a celebration of his unique perspective on life. He dreams of one day opening his own gallery, where he can not only display his work but also provide a platform for other autistic artists to share their creations.

Viktor's story is a powerful reminder of the importance of recognizing and nurturing the strengths of individuals with autism. His art serves as a bridge, connecting people to the beauty of neurodiversity and the incredible potential that lies within every person, regardless of their neurological differences.

In a world that often focuses on the challenges of autism, Viktor Bevanda's journey shines a light on the extraordinary gifts that can emerge when we embrace and support neuro-diversity. His art is a testament to the fact that autism is not a barrier to success but a different way of experiencing and contributing to the world.We beseech you at this juncture to stop reading this book, grab your computer or iphone, and scan the QR codes below in order to see and appreciate Viktor's artwork. It is so different that only by seeing it in color will you begin to understand why we gave so much time to this extraordinary individual.

TV News                    Art for Sale                    YouTube

*John Elder Robison*

## The Boy Who Ignited the Stage: An Autistic Teen's Journey with KISS

In the annals of rock and roll history, few bands have left as indelible a mark as KISS. Known for their electrifying performances, elaborate costumes, and, most notably, their groundbreaking use of pyrotechnics, KISS became legends of spectacle and sound. Behind one of the most iconic aspects of their stage shows was an unlikely contributor: an autistic teenager whose passion and ingenuity lit up the stage in more ways than one.

This remarkable story begins in the suburbs of New York City in the early 1970s, where a young boy named Johnny grew up with a fascination for fireworks and all things that sparkled and exploded. Not diagnosed with autism until age 40, Johnny often struggled with social interactions and traditional schooling. However, his parents noticed his extraordinary focus and technical prowess when it came to his hobbies, particularly his homemade pyrotechnic displays. His backyard experiments, though alarming to neighbors, showcased a natural talent and a meticulous attention to detail.

Johnny's father, a sound technician who occasionally worked with local bands, saw potential in his son's unusual skills. Through a series of fortunate connections, he managed to arrange a meeting with the members of KISS, who were then on the cusp of their rise to fame. Intrigued by the boy's enthusiasm and unique abilities, they decided to take a chance on him, despite his youth and unconventional background.

At just 16 years old, Johnny joined the KISS crew as an assistant, initially tasked with small, behind-the-scenes jobs. His keen eye for detail and unwavering dedication quickly caught the attention of the band and their production team. Johnny's autism, often seen as a challenge in other areas of his life, proved to be an asset in the high-pressure environment of live rock shows. His ability to hyper-focus allowed him to meticulously plan and execute complex pyrotechnic sequences with precision.

Over time, Johnny's role expanded. He began to design and implement larger and more intricate pyrotechnic displays, each show more dazzling than the last. The iconic fire-breathing, smoking guitars, and explosive stage effects that became synonymous with KISS were, in large part, a result of Johnny's creativity and technical expertise. His contributions transformed their concerts into unforgettable sensory experiences, thrilling audiences around the world.

Despite his growing responsibilities, Johnny remained humble and deeply committed to his work. He rarely sought the spotlight, content to let the band bask in the glory while he ensured every explosion, spark, and flame was executed perfectly. His autism, often misunderstood and stigmatized by society, found a unique and valuable expression through his work with KISS.

Johnny's story is not just one of personal triumph but also a testament to the power of inclusion and the untapped potential within every individual. His journey with KISS illustrates how embracing diversity and fostering unique talents can lead to groundbreaking innovation and success. Today, Johnny's legacy lives on in the countless bands and performers who have been inspired by his pioneering work in pyrotechnics.

In the world of rock and roll, where legends are born and spectacles are created, Johnny's tale is a shining example of how passion, perseverance, and a bit of fire can light up the world in the most unexpected ways. Of particular note is the book he wrote at a later age, "Look Me in the Eye" which is considered to be one of the first autobiographies ever written by a person with ASD. His book was a resounding success and can be found on Amazon books. You will not be disappointed if you purchase it.

*Other Lesser Known but Equally Talented Individuals*

Imagine a spectrum where every point of light is a story of achievement. On one end, there's Jonathan, a young man whose fascination with patterns led him to a brilliant career in mathematics, contributing to complex algorithms used in artificial intelligence. On the other, meet Sarah, an artist whose paintings, characterized by vibrant colors and intricate details, have found their way into esteemed galleries and have been a medium for her to communicate her inner world. Then there's Michael, a teenager with a penchant for athletics, who, despite his coordination challenges, has won several state-level swimming championships. And not to overlook Elena, who turned her meticulous nature into a successful entrepreneurial venture by starting a bakery that specializes in dietary-specific recipes, particularly catering to individuals with gluten sensitivities and other dietary restrictions.

Each of these individuals started their journey from different points but shared common hurdles: societal misconceptions, communication barriers, and sensory challenges. Yet, their stories converge on a triumphant note, underscoring the rich tapestry of potential that exists within the autism spectrum. These narratives emphasize that success in the autism community is as varied as the spectrum itself, reflecting a broad array of talents and abilities that flourish under the right conditions.

**Overcoming Obstacles**

The journey to success for many individuals with autism is often paved with significant obstacles. For Jonathan, the challenge was navigating the social dynamics of academic collaboration, a hurdle he overcame through dedicated social skills training and a supportive network of mentors and peers who recognized his potential and adapted their interactions to suit his communication style. Sarah had to contend with sensory overload in busy galleries. Her breakthrough came through the use of noise-canceling headphones and scheduled quiet hours, which allowed her to participate in exhibitions without overwhelming distress.

Michael's journey involved overcoming physical coordination difficulties, a feat achieved with the help of a coach who specialized in sports therapy for children with motor challenges. This tailored approach not only improved his athletic performance but also boosted his self-esteem and social standing among his peers. Elena faced initial skepticism about her business idea, but her meticulous attention to detail and the unique niche of her bakery quickly turned doubters into patrons and supporters.

## Role of Support Systems

None of these successes occurred in isolation. Behind each story is a robust support system comprising family, friends, educators, and sometimes, professionals who believed in their potential and provided the necessary support. Jonathan's university mentors adapted their teaching strategies, providing him with visual aids and one-on-one sessions. Sarah's family played a crucial role, creating a sensory-friendly workspace at home where she could paint in tranquility. Michael's coach and teammates cheered him on, providing both technical advice and moral support, while Elena's family assisted with the initial setup of her bakery, from finances to finding the right location.

These support systems were not merely aids; they were integral to each individual's success. They provided not just practical help but also emotional encouragement, understanding, and validation of their efforts and aspirations. This collective support underscores the importance of community and tailored interventions in nurturing the talents and abilities of individuals with autism.

## Impact of Early Intervention and Continuous Support

Reflecting on these stories, a common theme emerges: the critical role of early intervention and continuous support. Early diagnosis and tailored educational programs helped these individuals understand their strengths and challenges from a young age, setting the stage for appropriate interventions that catered to their developmental needs. For instance, early speech therapy and social skills training were pivotal in helping Jonathan enhance his communication skills, which later facilitated his academic collaborations.

Continuous support, adapting to each stage of their development, ensured that these individuals did not just cope with their challenges but thrived despite them. This ongoing support wasn't static; it evolved, recognizing that as these individuals grew, so too did their needs and aspirations. It's a testament to the enduring impact of sustained guidance and the adaptability of support systems to foster long-term success.

These narratives not only celebrate the achievements of individuals with autism but also serve as compelling evidence of the profound impact that understanding, support, and appropriate interventions can have on their lives. They remind us that with the right conditions, the potential for success is boundless, and the paths to achieving it are as diverse as the spectrum itself.

## 16.2 LESSONS LEARNED FROM FAMILIES LIVING WITH AUTISM

### Effective Communication Strategies

Navigating the complexities of autism within the family dynamic often hinges on effective communication. Many families have discovered that straightforward, consistent methods of communication can significantly enhance interactions and strengthen familial bonds. For instance, one family found that using clear, concise language and visual aids such as picture cards drastically reduced frustrations during daily routines for their non-verbal child. This method allowed the child to express needs and preferences without the stress of misunderstanding, fostering a calmer household environment.

Another strategy involves establishing a 'communication diary'—a shared notebook or digital document where family members jot down important daily happenings and feelings. This tool was particularly beneficial for a family with a teenager on the spectrum, who found face-to-face discussions overwhelming. The diary provided a space for him to articulate his thoughts and feelings at his own pace, improving family understanding and support. These communication techniques are not just about conveying messages; they are about building bridges, ensuring every family member feels heard and connected.

## Navigating Educational and Healthcare Systems

Families often encounter a maze of challenges within educational and healthcare systems, yet many have navigated these with notable success. One family shared their experience with securing the necessary educational accommodations for their daughter. They emphasized the importance of being well-prepared for Individualized Education Program (IEP) meetings, armed with comprehensive records of their child's needs and progress. Their proactive approach and persistent advocacy ensured their daughter received personalized support, setting a precedent for other families in similar situations.

Healthcare experiences shared by families underscore the importance of finding specialists who are knowledgeable about autism. One family recounted their journey across several states to find a pediatrician who specialized in developmental disorders, a decision that transformed their son's healthcare experience due to the specialist's deeper understanding of autism. These anecdotes highlight a crucial lesson: the relentless pursuit of appropriate and compassionate professional support is often necessary and invariably rewarding.

## Maintaining Family Balance

The challenge of maintaining balance and harmony in a family affected by autism is profound yet achievable. Families have shared that setting aside dedicated time for each family member is vital. For example, one family instituted a routine where each weekend, every family member, including the sibling without autism, chooses an activity. This practice ensures that everyone's interests and needs are honored, fostering a sense of inclusivity and preventing feelings of neglect.

Regular family meetings have also proven beneficial. These gatherings allow family members to express any concerns and discuss upcoming plans, ensuring everyone is on the same page. Such meetings reinforce the notion of teamwork and shared responsibility, which is crucial in a household where much attention might naturally gravitate towards the family member with autism.

### Community Involvement and Advocacy

Engagement in community advocacy and support networks stands out as not only transformative for the families involved but also immensely beneficial to the broader community. One family's initiative to start a local support group led to the development of an extensive network that advocates for city-wide policy changes to improve accessibility for individuals with autism. Their efforts have increased local awareness and prompted the implementation of autism-friendly public spaces.

Another family's involvement in autism workshops and seminars has empowered them to share their experiences and strategies, helping other families navigate similar challenges. Their active participation has created ripple effects, fostering a community environment that is more informed and inclusive.

These stories from families living with autism illuminate the profound impact of perseverance, creativity, and community engagement. They remind us that while the journey with autism is fraught with challenges, it is also replete with opportunities for growth, learning, and advocacy. Through shared experiences and collective wisdom, families continue to forge paths of support and understanding, contributing to a more inclusive and empathetic society.

As we close this chapter on family lessons, we carry forward the understanding that the journey with autism, though deeply personal, is interconnected with the broader tapestry of community life. The insights shared here pave the way for the subsequent discussions on advanced communication techniques, where we will explore how families can further enhance their communication strategies to support their loved ones with autism effectively.

# ADVANCED COMMUNICATION
# TECHNIQUES

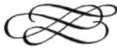

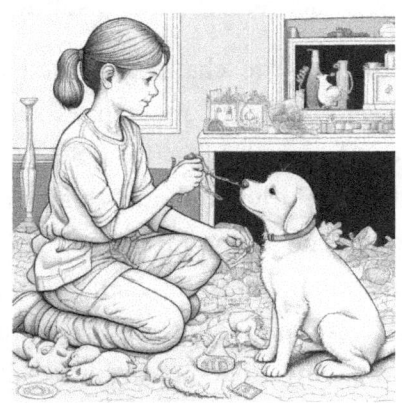

As your child matures into the complexities of teenage years, the way they communicate and understand the world evolves dramatically. During this transformative period, enhancing their communication skills becomes not just a supportive endeavor but a pivotal one. This chapter focuses on refining and expanding the communication abilities of older children with Autism Spectrum Disorder (ASD), which is crucial for their ability to express themselves and navigate the social intricacies of their environment.

## 17.1 ENHANCING COMMUNICATION WITH OLDER CHILDREN

### Developing Abstract Thinking

One of the milestones in the development of communication skills in older children with autism is the ability to understand and use abstract concepts. Abstract thinking is the capacity to process ideas that are not directly tied to concrete physical experiences—concepts such as metaphorical thinking, idioms, and humor. This form of thinking is crucial because much of everyday language and social interaction relies on abstract references and subtle cues.

For instance, consider the challenge posed by idioms like "It's raining cats and dogs" or metaphors such as "He has a heart of stone." To a child with ASD, these could be confusing if taken literally. To aid in this area, one effective method is through metaphor interpretation exercises. You can start by introducing simple metaphors and gradually progress to more complex ones, discussing and explaining the underlying meanings together. Additionally, using visual aids like cartoons or storyboards can help illustrate these concepts more concretely.

Another interactive way to develop abstract thinking is through humor exercises, which can be both engaging and educational. Initiating playful banter or introducing age-appropriate jokes allows your child to explore the nuances of language and expressions used in humor. This not only aids in linguistic development but also enhances social bonding.

**Expanding Vocabulary and Concepts**

As children grow, so too should their vocabulary and the concepts they understand. This expansion is vital not only for academic success but also for everyday interactions and personal expression. Engaging in thematic learning is a beneficial strategy here. For example, if your child shows interest in space, you can explore this theme across different subjects—science (learning about planets), literature (reading stories about space travel), and even art (creating spaceship models).

Utilizing multimedia resources can also be incredibly effective. Educational videos, interactive games, and audiobooks can introduce new vocabulary in a dynamic and engaging context, making the learning process more enjoyable and memorable. Moreover, regular discussions on diverse topics can challenge your child's understanding and encourage them to express their thoughts and opinions, thereby practicing newly acquired words and phrases.

**Facilitating Multimodal Communication**

Communication is not just about words; it involves a symphony of verbal, non-verbal, and written cues. Older children with autism can benefit significantly from learning how to integrate these different modes of communication effectively. For instance, while discussing a topic, encourage your child to express what they feel not just through words but also through facial expressions or even drawing. This practice helps them understand that communication is multifaceted and that different situations may require different methods of expression.

Modeling multimodal communication yourself can be a powerful teaching tool. Demonstrate how tone of voice can affect the meaning of a sentence or how eye contact can convey sincerity. Through such modeling, you provide your child with clear examples to emulate, which can be particularly helpful in teaching subtle aspects of communication that are often taken for granted.

**Role-Playing and Scenario-Based Practice**

Role-playing is an excellent method for practicing and mastering complex conversations and social interactions that your child is likely to encounter. Create scenarios that they might face, such as interacting with a bank teller, going on a date, or handling a job interview. These role-playing sessions can allow your child to practice responses and behaviors in a safe and supportive environment before they encounter these situations in real life.

For each scenario, discuss possible variations in conversations and encourage your child to think about and respond to different outcomes. This not only prepares them for the specific situation but also enhances their ability to think on their feet and adapt to changing social dynamics. Over time, these practice sessions build confidence and reduce anxiety about real-world interactions, empowering your child to navigate the social world more effectively.

**Interactive Element: Role-Playing Activity Guide**

To facilitate the incorporation of role-playing into your communication practice routines, here is a structured guide to setting up effective role-playing exercises:

- Choose a Scenario: Select a common social situation your child might encounter that involves complex communication or social norms.
- Define Roles: Clearly define the roles involved in the scenario. You can take one role, and your child takes another, or use siblings or friends in the role-play.
- Set Objectives: Determine what communication skills or social norms you want to focus on. For instance, you might focus on polite requesting, expressing disagreement respectfully, or maintaining eye contact.
- Prepare Props: Use props where necessary to make the scenario more realistic. Props can be as simple as a table and chairs to simulate a dining scenario or paper money for a buying and selling interaction.
- Practice and Switch Roles: Allow your child to practice the scenario multiple times, possibly switching roles to see the situation from different perspectives.
- Discuss and Reflect: After the role-play, discuss what went well and what could be improved. Encourage your child to express how they felt during the scenario and reflect on the effectiveness of their communication.

This activity guide is designed to make role-playing a fun and educational tool for enhancing communication skills in older children with ASD, providing them with the confidence and competence to handle complex social interactions.

## 17.2 ADVANCED SOCIAL CUES UNDERSTANDING FOR ADULTS ON THE SPECTRUM

Navigating the nuanced landscape of social interactions can pose significant challenges for adults with Autism Spectrum Disorder (ASD), particularly as they decode complex social cues like sarcasm, indirect language, and concealed emotions. These subtleties of communication often go unnoticed or misunderstood by individuals on the spectrum, making everyday interactions feel like navigating a maze without a map. To enhance understanding and mastery of these social cues, several strategies and tools can be employed effectively.

Social stories are a powerful educational tool that can help in breaking down the components of complex social interactions into understandable parts. These stories simplify social situations and explain them step-by-step, making it easier for adults with ASD to grasp the underlying concepts of sarcasm or indirect requests. For instance, a social story about a co-worker saying, "Great weather we're having!" during a storm can illustrate the use of sarcasm, explaining that the co-worker doesn't literally mean what they're saying. Additionally, video modeling can serve as a visual guide by showing scenarios where sarcasm or indirect language is used, accompanied by explanations of the context and the appropriate responses. These videos can be reviewed multiple times, helping to reinforce learning and understanding.

Real-time feedback is another crucial element in learning to interpret complex social cues. This involves receiving immediate correction or confirmation during actual social interactions, which can help in making the necessary adjustments to one's behavior or understanding in the moment. For example, if an adult with ASD responds too literally to a sarcastic comment, a trusted friend or mentor can gently explain the actual intent of the comment, helping to clarify misunderstandings as they occur. This immediate feedback helps integrate the learning directly into real-life situations, making it more applicable and accessible.

In professional environments, adults with ASD often face unique communication challenges that can impact their work relationships and career progression. Understanding workplace norms, engaging in small talk, and handling criticism are essential skills for professional success. Strategies to navigate these challenges include explicit training on workplace etiquette, which can outline the expectations and unwritten rules of office culture. For engaging in small talk, practicing set phrases or topics in advance can provide a safety net, allowing the individual to feel prepared and less anxious about spontaneous conversations. Additionally, handling professional criticism constructively can be facilitated through role-plays or scenarios where feedback is given and received, helping to desensitize and educate on appropriate responses.

Empathetic listening and responding are integral to building and maintaining relationships. This skill involves more than just hearing words; it requires understanding the emotions and intentions behind them. Techniques to enhance empathetic listening include exercises that focus on recognizing emotional expressions and understanding different perspectives. For instance, watching films or reading books and discussing the characters' emotions and motivations can be a useful exercise. Practicing active listening, where the listener reflects back what they've heard and asks questions to clarify, also strengthens this skill.

Technological tools offer additional support for mastering social cues. Virtual reality (VR) environments can simulate social interactions in a controlled setting, allowing for practice without the real-world consequences of misunderstandings. Apps designed to train facial recognition and emotional interpretation can provide regular exercises to improve the ability to read and respond to non-verbal cues. Online platforms that offer structured social skills training can also be beneficial, providing resources and community support to practice and refine these skills.

By leveraging these tools and strategies, adults with ASD can enhance their ability to understand and interact within the social world more effectively. The journey toward mastering complex social cues is continuous, but with the right support, significant progress can be made.

As we conclude this exploration of advanced communication techniques for adults with ASD, we recognize the profound impact that improved social understanding can have on an individual's personal and professional life. Through dedicated practice and the integration of supportive tools and strategies, adults on the spectrum can enhance their communication skills, leading to more meaningful interactions and opportunities. The next chapter will build on these foundations by delving into the challenges and strategies associated with therapy and intervention, aiming to provide a holistic approach to supporting adults with ASD in all aspects of life.

# THERAPY AND INTERVENTION

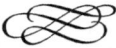

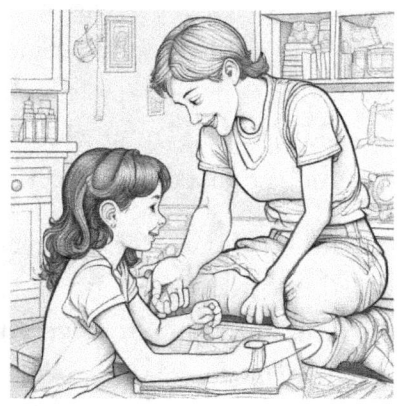

Navigating the landscape of therapeutic interventions for Autism Spectrum Disorder (ASD) can often feel as complex and varied as the spectrum itself. Each child is unique, and as such, the therapies that resonate and yield the most significant benefits can vary dramatically from one individual to another. In this chapter, we will explore the gamut of therapeutic options available, from well-established practices to innovative and emerging therapies, providing you with the insights needed to make informed choices for your child.

## 18.1 OVERVIEW OF THERAPEUTIC MODALITIES FOR AUTISM

### Introduction to Common Therapies

In the realm of autism therapy, several key modalities form the backbone of treatment strategies. Among these, Applied Behavior Analysis (ABA) stands out as one of the most researched and widely adopted approaches. ABA is primarily focused on improving specific behaviors, including social skills, communication, reading, and academics, through reinforcement strategies. This therapy is highly data-driven, allowing for detailed tracking of a child's progress and tailoring of interventions to maximize effectiveness.

Occupational Therapy (OT) is another cornerstone in autism treatment, aimed at enhancing daily living skills. OT helps children develop skills necessary for everyday tasks from dressing and eating to more complex skills like problem-solving and time management. The therapy is often customized to address sensory integration issues, a common challenge for many on the spectrum, helping them process sensory information more effectively.

Speech Therapy is crucial for those with speech and language difficulties, a common trait associated with autism. This therapy focuses on improving verbal, nonverbal, and social communication. Techniques might include articulation therapy, language intervention activities, and others such as the Picture Exchange Communication System (PECS) for those who are non-verbal.

Social Skills Therapy is dedicated to improving an individual's ability to interact with others effectively. This often involves group sessions where children can practice social skills in a structured environment under the guidance of a therapist, learning everything from sharing and taking turns to understanding body language and facial expressions.

**Emerging Therapies**

Beyond these traditional approaches, several emerging therapies are gaining traction within the autism community for their innovative methods and promising results. Music Therapy, for instance, uses music as a therapeutic tool to address physical, emotional, cognitive, and social needs of individuals. It can enhance communication, attention, and emotional regulation in ways that are engaging and enjoyable for the child.

Art Therapy allows individuals with ASD to express themselves and process complex feelings through creative mediums like drawing, painting, or sculpting. This form of therapy can be particularly beneficial for those who find verbal communication challenging, providing a visual mode of expression that can be more accessible and revealing. In case you missed it, please go back to Chapter 16 and scan the QR code marked "YouTube" where you can see Vicktor Bevanda's incredible art skills along with his limited verbal skills.

Equine Therapy involves interactions with horses under the guidance of a professional therapist to help improve a range of emotional and physical skills. The rhythmic nature of horse riding and the necessity to engage with a responsive animal can improve motor skills, coordination, and emotional bonding patterns. Besides horses, we have found children with ASD bond very strongly with dogs as well. They will spend hours talking to their dog at the same time completely neglecting the adults or parents in the room.

## Integrative Approach to Therapy

The integrative approach in autism therapy is a holistic strategy that combines elements from various therapies to address the multifaceted needs of individuals with autism. This method acknowledges that no single therapy can comprehensively address all aspects of autism and that combining approaches can lead to more significant improvements across different areas of development.

For example, a child might engage in both ABA for behavioral improvements and OT for sensory integration, along with Speech Therapy to enhance communication skills. This integrated approach ensures that therapeutic interventions are well-rounded, addressing various dimensions of the child's development simultaneously.

## Family Involvement in Therapies

The role of the family in the therapeutic process cannot be overstated. Your involvement as a parent or caregiver is crucial in reinforcing the gains made during therapy sessions and in ensuring consistency and continuity in interventions. Engaging in therapy sessions, when appropriate, can help you understand the techniques used by therapists, allowing you to replicate these strategies at home.

Moreover, your support and reinforcement outside of therapy sessions can significantly influence the effectiveness of the treatments. Being involved gives you insights into your child's progress, challenges, and responds to different therapies, which is invaluable in tailoring interventions to meet their evolving needs.

**Interactive Element: Case Study Reflection**

To further illustrate the impact of an integrative approach combined with family involvement, let's consider a case study:

- Case Study: Emma, a 7-year-old girl with ASD, engaged in a combination of ABA, OT, and Speech Therapy. Her parents participated in training sessions to learn specific strategies used during her therapies. At home, they created a supportive environment that mirrored her therapy sessions, using visual schedules and reward systems similar to those used by her ABA therapist, and sensory integration tools recommended by her occupational therapist. Over six months, Emma showed significant improvements in her communication abilities, sensory processing, and behavioral responses.

This case highlights the synergy between multiple therapeutic modalities and active family involvement, underscoring the potential for enhanced outcomes when these elements are effectively combined.

## 18.2 EVALUATING THE EFFECTIVENESS OF DIFFERENT THERAPIES

When you embark on a therapeutic path for your child with Autism Spectrum Disorder, it's crucial to assess the effectiveness of the treatments to ensure they are meeting your child's needs. One fundamental way to gauge this is by establishing specific criteria that reflect measurable changes and improvements in your child's abilities and behaviors. For instance, you might look for advancements in communication skills, which could range from increased verbal outputs to more complex conversational exchanges. Similarly, a reduction in problematic behaviors such as outbursts or repetitive actions, or an enhancement in social interactions like initiating play with peers, can serve as clear indicators of a therapy's impact.

Setting measurable goals is vital for this evaluation process. These goals should be specific, measurable, achievable, relevant, and time-bound (SMART), tailored to your child's individual challenges and strengths. For example, if your child struggles with verbal communication, a goal might be for them to initiate conversation at least once during therapy sessions within a three-month period. Regular monitoring and progress tracking are essential in this context, providing a clear view of whether the interventions are yielding the desired outcomes. This ongoing assessment not only helps in recognizing successes but also in identifying areas where adjustments might be needed.

Personalizing therapy plans is another critical aspect of effective treatment. Autism manifests uniquely in each individual; thus, therapeutic approaches must be equally unique to cater to these diverse needs. Factors such as the child's age, the severity and spectrum of their symptoms, and their personal interests should influence the customization of therapy plans. For a younger child with mild sensory issues, for instance, occupational therapy might focus more on play-based activities that integrate sensory integration techniques. For an older child with significant social communication deficits, a combination of speech therapy and social skills groups might be more appropriate. The key is to align therapeutic methods with the child's developmental stage and personal affinities, which can significantly boost engagement and outcomes.

The role of continuous feedback in therapy cannot be overstated. Effective therapy requires an adaptive approach that responds to the child's evolving needs. Regular feedback sessions with therapists provide insights into progress and challenges, forming the basis for necessary adjustments to the therapy regimen. This might mean increasing the intensity of interventions, introducing new techniques, or even phasing out therapies that are no longer beneficial. Collaborative decision-making, involving therapists, parents, and sometimes even the child, depending on their age and cognitive ability, ensures that adjustments to the therapy plan are informed, thoughtful, and tailored to ongoing developmental shifts.

Lastly, the foundation of any therapeutic approach should be built on solid scientific research and evidence. Well-established therapies like Applied Behavior Analysis (ABA) have a robust body of research supporting their efficacy in improving specific behaviors in autism. However, newer modalities like art therapy or technology-assisted interventions are also showing promise according to recent studies. Staying informed about the latest research and evidence not only assists in choosing the right therapies but also in understanding the mechanisms behind their effectiveness. This knowledge empowers you to make informed decisions about your child's treatment plan, ensuring it is supported by the best available evidence.

As you navigate the complexities of autism therapies, remember that the goal is to find the most effective strategies that empower your child to reach their full potential. By evaluating therapies against clear criteria, personalizing interventions, adapting to feedback, and grounding decisions in solid research, you can ensure that the therapeutic journey is as productive and positive as it can be.

In concluding this chapter, we've explored the multifaceted approach to evaluating and optimizing therapies for children with autism. This process is crucial not just for immediate developmental gains but also for setting the stage for long-term growth and independence. As we transition to the next chapter, we will delve into future trends in autism research and treatment, providing a glimpse into innovative developments that continue to shape our understanding and management of autism.

# FUTURE TRENDS IN AUTISM RESEARCH AND TREATMENT

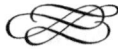

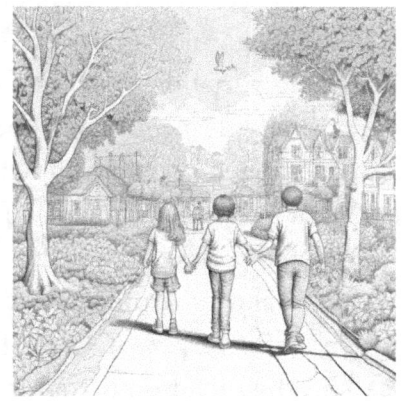

As we peer into the evolving landscape of autism research and treatment, it becomes evident that the future holds promising advancements that could fundamentally transform our approach to understanding and managing Autism Spectrum Disorder (ASD). These innovations are not just refining existing methodologies but are paving the way for groundbreaking changes in how we diagnose, interact with, and support individuals with autism. This chapter delves into some of the most exciting developments on the horizon, offering you a glimpse into the future of autism care that is informed by cutting-edge research and enhanced by technological breakthroughs.

## 19.1 CUTTING-EDGE RESEARCH IN AUTISM: WHAT'S ON THE HORIZON?

### Genetic and Neurological Studies

One of the most dynamic areas of autism research involves genetic and neurological studies which seek to unravel the intricate web of factors that contribute to the development of ASD. Recent advances in genetic technologies, such as whole-genome sequencing, have allowed researchers to identify specific genetic variations associated with autism. These studies are not only deepening our understanding of the complex genetic architecture of autism but are also highlighting the significant role environmental factors play in influencing these genetic risks. The interplay between genetic predispositions and environmental factors such as prenatal exposure to toxins or parental age at conception is becoming clearer, shedding light on the multifaceted nature of autism.

This burgeoning area of research holds the promise of developing more personalized approaches to treatment. By understanding an individual's specific genetic profile, clinicians could tailor interventions that are more effective and have fewer side effects, moving away from the one-size-fits-all approach that often prevails in treatment plans today. Imagine a future where treatment can be customized not just to the symptoms of ASD but to the underlying genetic factors contributing to these symptoms, potentially enhancing outcomes significantly.

## Early Detection and Intervention

In the realm of early detection, researchers are making significant strides in identifying markers of autism earlier in a child's development, well before traditional behavioral symptoms become apparent. Innovations in screening tools, which now include the analysis of eye tracking patterns, vocalizations, and even fine motor movements, are proving to be promising in identifying ASD at a much younger age. Early diagnosis is pivotal as it opens the door to early intervention, which can profoundly impact a child's developmental trajectory.

Timely and effective interventions can enhance cognitive, language, and social skills, thereby improving long-term outcomes in education, employment, and social integration. The potential of these early interventions to modify the course of autism development highlights the critical importance of ongoing research and development in early diagnostic tools.

## Cognitive and Behavioral Models

As our understanding of autism deepens, new cognitive and behavioral models are emerging that offer fresh insights into the diverse manifestations of ASD. These models are crucial for developing targeted therapies that address the specific challenges faced by individuals with autism. By refining our understanding of how cognitive processes like attention, perception, and problem-solving differ in individuals with ASD, therapists can better tailor their approaches to meet these unique needs.

Moreover, these advanced models are guiding the development of specialized educational programs and behavioral interventions that are more aligned with the cognitive profiles of individuals with autism. This tailored approach not only enhances the effectiveness of interventions but also supports a higher degree of personalization in treatment plans.

**Technology-Enhanced Therapies**

Perhaps one of the most transformative trends in autism research and treatment is the integration of technology. Innovative uses of virtual reality (VR) and augmented reality (AR) are revolutionizing social skills training by providing immersive, interactive environments where individuals with autism can practice and refine social interactions in a controlled, repeatable manner. These technologies offer safe spaces for experimentation without the fear of real-world consequences, making them ideal tools for individuals on the spectrum.

Additionally, AI-driven diagnostic tools and therapeutic aids are being developed to provide real-time, data-driven insights into the effectiveness of various interventions. These technologies not only enhance the precision of treatments but also make therapeutic tools more accessible to families who might not have ready access to specialized care. The potential for these technologies to democratize access to high-quality interventions is just beginning to be tapped.

In this rapidly evolving field, the conjunction of research and technology is setting the stage for a future where the nuances of autism are not just better understood but more effectively addressed. As we continue to explore these promising avenues, the potential to improve the quality of life for individuals with autism and their families expands dramatically, heralding a future that is more inclusive and empowering for all involved.

## 19.2 INNOVATIONS IN TREATMENT AND CARE

**Integrative Health Approaches**

The landscape of autism treatment is witnessing a significant shift towards integrative health approaches, a trend that marries traditional therapies with complementary practices such as nutrition, physical exercise, and mindfulness. This holistic view of treatment recognizes that the challenges of autism spectrum disorder (ASD) are multifaceted, affecting not just cognitive and behavioral dimensions, but also physical and emotional health. Nutrition, for instance, plays a critical role in managing ASD, with certain dietary adjustments often leading to improvements in behavior and cognitive function. Incorporating a balanced diet rich in nutrients can mitigate common digestive issues associated with autism and improve overall well-being.

Physical exercise, too, is more than just a health requirement; for individuals with autism, it can serve as a powerful tool for improving motor skills, reducing anxiety, and enhancing mood. Structured physical activities like yoga or team sports are not only avenues for physical health but also social interaction and the development of teamwork skills. Meanwhile, mindfulness practices such as meditation and controlled breathing can significantly improve concentration, sleep, and emotional regulation, helping individuals with ASD cope with anxiety and sensory overload. These integrative approaches are gaining traction because they offer a more comprehensive treatment model that acknowledges and addresses the complex needs of individuals with autism, enhancing their quality of life and long-term outcomes.

## Community-Based Models

Community-based treatment models are transforming the support landscape for individuals with autism by fostering inclusivity and providing holistic support. These models integrate various services—education, healthcare, and community activities—into a cohesive framework that supports individuals with autism throughout their life span. For example, some communities have developed inclusive educational programs that not only cater to students with autism but also educate their neurotypical peers about diversity and inclusion, fostering a supportive school environment.

Healthcare services in these models are coordinated to ensure that individuals with autism receive comprehensive care that extends beyond medical treatment to include occupational therapy, speech therapy, and mental health services. Additionally, community activities are designed to be accessible and enjoyable for individuals with autism, providing them with opportunities to engage with the community, pursue their interests, and form social connections. These community-based models are crucial because they create ecosystems of support that understand and cater to the needs of individuals with autism, enabling them to lead fulfilling lives.

## Patient-Centered Care Innovations

Innovations in patient-centered care are crucial in transforming the treatment and management of autism by putting the preferences and insights of individuals with autism at the forefront of care decisions. This approach involves patients more directly in their treatment plans, respecting their input and adjusting interventions accordingly. Such inclusivity can significantly enhance satisfaction with care and improve treatment outcomes. For instance, some clinics now use tools that allow patients with autism to communicate their preferences and discomforts effectively, which helps medical professionals tailor their approaches in real-time to suit individual needs.

Moreover, patient-centered care often involves families and caregivers to a greater extent, ensuring that the strategies developed are practical and sustainable across home and clinical settings. By respecting the voices of those with autism and considering their lived experiences in treatment plans, healthcare providers can deliver more effective, compassionate, and personalized care.

## Global Collaboration in Autism Research and Treatment

The global collaboration in autism research and treatment is playing a pivotal role in harmonizing approaches and sharing successful practices across borders. International research collaborations are pooling resources and expertise to tackle complex questions about autism more effectively, leading to faster and more robust findings. For example, multinational studies are exploring the genetic foundations of autism, providing insights that transcend individual populations and contribute to a global understanding of the disorder.

Furthermore, global educational and healthcare initiatives are sharing successful intervention strategies and training materials, ensuring that effective treatment methods are accessible worldwide. These collaborations are particularly beneficial for countries with less developed autism support infrastructures, as they can adopt and adapt proven strategies and tools. By fostering international cooperation, the global autism community is working towards a future where effective, compassionate care and support for individuals with autism are available regardless of geographical location.

As we conclude this exploration of the latest innovations in autism treatment and care, we see a promising horizon enriched by holistic health models, community support systems, patient-centered care approaches, and international collaborations. These developments are not just advancing our capabilities in treating autism but are fundamentally changing how we think about and interact with individuals on the spectrum. As we move into the next chapter, we will delve into creating a legacy of understanding and support that transcends generations, aiming for a future where individuals with autism are fully integrated and active participants in all aspects of life.

# CREATING A LEGACY OF
# UNDERSTANDING

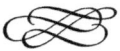

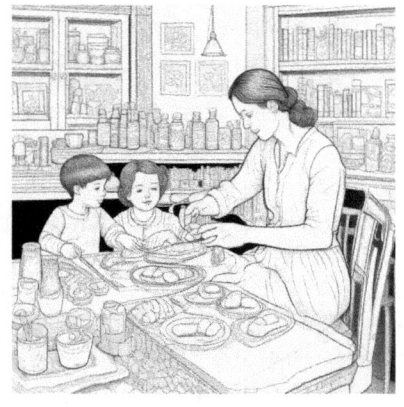

Imagine, for a moment, the profound impact your experiences could have on others navigating the complex world of Autism Spectrum Disorder (ASD). Each challenge you've faced, each victory you've celebrated, holds invaluable lessons not just for you but for the countless others who might be at the beginning of their path or somewhere along its winding course. This chapter aims to equip you with the tools and insights necessary to transform your peronsider roles that align with your skills and interests. If you are an organized person, you might coordinate support group meetings or fundraising events. If you have a knack for education, you might facilitate workshops or informational sessions. Your involvement can bring new energy and perspectives to these initiatives, driving forward the mission to support and empower individuals with ASD and their families.

**Creating Educational Materials**

Your insights and practical knowledge gained from firsthand experience are invaluable educational tools for others. Developing resources such as pamphlets, videos, or interactive workshops allows you to distill complex information into accessible formats that can benefit educators, parents, and even policymakers.

For instance, creating a video series that offers tips on daily living activities or social skills can be a significant aid for other families. These materials should be clear, concise, and infused with empathy and understanding, reflecting the realities of living with ASD while providing practical advice and encouragement.

**Mentoring and Support**

Mentoring is perhaps one of the most direct ways to support others on their autism journey. As a mentor, you can provide guidance, share resources, and offer emotional support to families adjusting to a new diagnosis or navigating particular challenges associated with ASD. This relationship can be incredibly rewarding and transformative, not just for the mentee but for you as well.

When acting as a mentor, it's vital to listen actively, provide tailored advice based on your experiences, and always respect the unique perspectives and choices of the mentee's family. Your role is not to dictate but to guide and support, helping others find their path through the complexities of ASD with greater confidence and less isolation.

Weave your personal journey into a beacon of hope and guidance for others. By sharing your story, volunteering your time, creating educational materials, and offering mentorship, you can extend a hand to those who are just starting to find their way.

## 20.1 HOW TO USE YOUR EXPERIENCE TO HELP OTHERS

**Sharing Your Story**

The power of personal narratives in shaping perceptions and understanding cannot be overstated. Your journey with autism is a narrative of unique challenges and triumphs, a story that when shared, can profoundly touch the hearts and minds of others. Whether through blog posts, social media platforms, or speaking engagements, articulating your experiences can demystify aspects of ASD, offer practical insights, and foster a deeper sense of empathy and community among those affected by autism. Watching the YouTube video (the right hand QR code at the end of Chapter 16) of Viktor Bevanda provides us all with an insight into the handicaps a child with ASD can have, and yet at the same time exemplifies the incredible talent of that same child.

When preparing to share your story, consider the mediums that best match your comfort level and reach your intended audience effectively. Blogs and social media offer platforms for ongoing dialogue and community building, while speaking engagements allow for more personal interaction and immediate feedback. It's important to be honest and open, yet mindful of how personal details about your family and your child are presented. Remember, each shared experience can become a lifeline of support and a source of comfort to someone feeling isolated in their struggles.

**Volunteering and Community Involvement**

Engaging directly with autism communities through volunteering is another powerful way to leverage your experience. Many organizations and support groups thrive on the dedication of volunteers who organize events, run programs, and provide direct support to families. By volunteering, you not only enrich the lives of others but also strengthen your own understanding of ASD, staying informed about new research and emerging resources.

By sharing your story, volunteering your time, creating educational materials, and mentoring others, you are not just passing on knowledge—you are fostering a community bound by understanding and support. Through these actions, you contribute to a legacy of empathy, resilience, and collective empowerment that will resonate within the autism community for generations to come.

## 20.2 ADVOCATING FOR CHANGE IN PUBLIC PERCEPTION OF AUTISM

When discussing the impact of autism on a family, it's crucial to consider how societal perceptions and misconceptions can profoundly shape experiences. Each interaction in the public sphere presents an opportunity to educate and influence, to reshape understanding and encourage a more inclusive and supportive community. Addressing these misconceptions requires a strategic approach, one that involves clear communication, engagement with the media, active policy advocacy, and direct outreach through educational presentations.

### Addressing Misconceptions

Misconceptions about autism are widespread, ranging from stereotypes about the capabilities of individuals with ASD to misunderstandings about the causes of the disorder. To counter these, it's essential to engage in open conversations where misinformation can be corrected. This could involve speaking up in social settings, writing informative posts online, or participating in community discussions. The key is to provide accurate information and share personal experiences that highlight the diversity and capabilities of individuals with autism. These conversations often require patience and empathy, as changing deep-seated beliefs doesn't happen overnight. By consistently presenting facts and personal stories, you can help dismantle myths and foster a deeper understanding of autism.

## Media Engagement

The media plays a pivotal role in shaping public perception, making it a powerful platform for advocacy. Engaging with the media can range from writing opinion pieces (op-eds) for newspapers or magazines to participating in interviews or podcast discussions about autism. These opportunities allow you to reach a broader audience, spreading awareness and promoting a more accurate depiction of autism. When engaging with the media, it's beneficial to prepare key messages beforehand to ensure clarity and impact. Additionally, collaborating with autism advocacy organizations can amplify your voice, providing a unified front that can push for greater changes in media representation of autism.

## Policy Advocacy

Advocating for policy changes is another crucial aspect of transforming public perception and creating a supportive environment for individuals with autism. This can involve several strategies, such as connecting with legislators, participating in hearings, or joining advocacy networks that focus on disability rights. When advocating for policy change, it's important to be well-informed about the issues at hand and the specific changes you wish to see implemented. Preparing position papers, gathering community support, and organizing meetings with policymakers are all effective ways to influence autism-related policies. Additionally, attending public forums and using these platforms to speak about autism can raise public and legislative awareness, driving home the need for policies that support inclusion and accessibility.

## School and Community Presentations

One of the most direct ways to educate others about autism is through presentations in schools and community centers. These presentations can be tailored to educate teachers, students, parents, and community members about the realities of autism, focusing on understanding, acceptance, and how to support individuals with autism in various settings. When organizing these presentations, it's useful to include interactive elements such as Q&A sessions, which encourage engagement and allow for a deeper exploration of the topics discussed. Additionally, involving individuals with autism to share their experiences can make these presentations more impactful, providing firsthand insights into the challenges and triumphs of living with autism.

Through these multifaceted advocacy efforts, you have the power to influence how autism is viewed and treated in society. By addressing misconceptions, engaging with the media, advocating for policy changes, and educating communities, you contribute to a more informed and compassionate world where individuals with autism can thrive.

## 20.3 SETTING REALISTIC GOALS AND CELEBRATING MILESTONES

Navigating through the complexities of raising a child with Autism Spectrum Disorder (ASD) requires not only patience and understanding but also a strategic approach to setting goals that are both realistic and achievable. When you consider your child's strengths and challenges, you can craft goals that promote growth while also respecting their unique pace and abilities. The art of goal-setting in the context of autism involves breaking larger objectives into smaller, manageable steps that can gradually build your child's skills and confidence. For instance, if the goal is to improve communication, you might start with nonverbal cues like pointing or using picture cards, gradually moving towards forming simple words and sentences as your child becomes more comfortable and capable.

This approach ensures that each step is within reach, preventing feelings of frustration and boosting morale both for you and your child. It is crucial to maintain flexibility in your goals, understanding that progress is not always linear and that adjustments may be necessary as your child grows and develops. Regular assessments can help you fine-tune these goals, ensuring they remain aligned with your child's evolving needs and capabilities. Moreover, involving your child in the goal-setting process can be incredibly empowering for them. It allows them to have a say in their own growth and contributes to a deeper sense of accomplishment as they achieve each milestone.

The celebration of milestones plays a central role in nurturing your child's self-esteem and motivation. Recognizing and celebrating every achievement, no matter how small, reinforces their efforts and encourages them to keep progressing. Simple acknowledgments like a sticker chart, a small treat, or a verbal praise can make a significant impact. These celebrations not only make your child feel valued and appreciated but also highlight the positive aspects of learning and development, making the process enjoyable and fulfilling for the whole family.

Documenting progress is another essential aspect of this journey. Keeping a journal, maintaining a portfolio of your child's work, or creating video logs can help track the improvements over time, providing a tangible way to see how far your child has come. These records serve as a motivational tool for both the child and the family, reminding everyone of the progress made and the hurdles overcome. They also offer valuable insights when planning future goals, allowing you to tailor your strategies based on what has been effective in the past.

As your child matures, the nature and scope of the goals will inevitably change. It's important to recognize when certain goals no longer serve their purpose and need modification. This adaptive approach not only keeps your strategies relevant but also ensures that they continue to challenge and engage your child appropriately. Adjusting goals isn't a sign of setback but rather an indication of your responsive and attuned parenting, which is crucial in meeting the ever-changing needs of a child with ASD. As you continue to guide your child through these developmental phases, remember that each small step contributes to a larger picture of growth and independence, crafting a fulfilling life experience for your child and the entire family.

## 20.4 UNDERSTANDING AND MANAGING ANXIETY IN AUTISTIC CHILDREN

Anxiety is not uncommon in children with Autism Spectrum Disorder (ASD), but it often manifests differently than it might in neurotypical children, making it crucial for you, as a parent, to recognize the unique signs in your child. Children with ASD may not always be able to express their feelings of anxiety verbally. Instead, signs of anxiety might appear as an increase in repetitive behaviors, disruptions in sleep patterns, or even physical symptoms like gastrointestinal distress. Understanding these cues is the first step in effectively managing anxiety, ensuring that your child can feel safer and more secure in their day-to-day interactions.

One effective strategy to manage anxiety involves the use of sensory integration techniques. Children with ASD often have sensory sensitivities that can contribute to their anxiety. By creating a sensory-friendly environment at home and school, you can help minimize these triggers. This might include dimming lights, reducing background noise, or providing tactile toys that can help soothe and calm. Additionally, structured routines can significantly reduce anxiety by providing predictability and a sense of control. Keeping a consistent schedule, with regular times for meals, school, therapy, and leisure activities can help create a stable environment that reduces uncertainty.

Relaxation exercises are also invaluable tools for managing anxiety. Techniques such as deep breathing, progressive muscle relaxation, or guided imagery can be taught and practiced routinely during calm periods so that your child can more readily draw upon them during stressful situations. Mindfulness activities, particularly those designed for children, such as simple yoga poses or mindfulness coloring, can be integrated into your child's daily routines, helping them to cultivate a state of awareness and calm from a young age.

## Professional Support Options

Knowing when and how to seek professional help is crucial in managing your child's anxiety effectively. Cognitive-behavioral therapy (CBT), for instance, has been adapted for children with ASD and can be particularly effective in helping them understand and manage their anxiety. CBT for autistic children often involves more visual aids and concrete examples and focuses on teaching skills through repetition and reinforcement. If you notice that your child's anxiety is impeding their ability to function or enjoy life, it may be time to consult with a professional who has experience in working with children with ASD.

When selecting a therapist, look for professionals who specialize in pediatric anxiety and have experience with children on the autism spectrum. It's important that they use evidence-based practices and are able to adapt these to meet the unique needs of your child. In some cases, medication may also be considered as part of a broader treatment plan. A developmental pediatrician, child psychiatrist, or a pediatric neurologist can guide you through the benefits and considerations of such treatments based on a thorough assessment of your child's specific needs.

## Creating a Supportive Environment

The environment in which your child lives and learns plays a pivotal role in managing their anxiety. A supportive home environment is one that anticipates potential anxiety triggers and has strategies in place to manage them. This might involve creating quiet spaces where your child can retreat when feeling overwhelmed or having a series of pre-planned activities that can serve as distractions during high-stress periods. Safety, predictability, and a sense of control are key elements in such environments.

Moreover, fostering open communication within the family about each person's needs and feelings can also help in managing anxiety. Encourage all family members to share their thoughts and concerns regularly. This not only helps in understanding each other better but also models healthy ways of expressing emotions and managing stress for your child.

By implementing these strategies, you equip your child with the tools they need to manage their anxiety more effectively. Regular practice of these techniques, combined with professional guidance when necessary, will help your child to navigate their world with less anxiety and more confidence. As they learn to manage their anxiety, they also gain skills that will serve them throughout their life, enhancing their overall well-being and ability to engage with the world around them.

## 20.5 THE IMPORTANCE OF ROUTINE IN AUTISTIC CHILDREN'S LIVES

Routines are the scaffolding of daily life, especially for children with Autism Spectrum Disorder (ASD). These structured frameworks are not merely about keeping a schedule; they serve as essential tools that imbue a child's world with predictability and security. For children with ASD, who often find the unpredictable nature of daily life challenging, routines can significantly reduce stress. They provide a predictable sequence of events that help these children navigate their day with less anxiety, understanding what comes next and what is expected of them. Moreover, routines can help enhance learning and behavior management by systematically integrating therapeutic activities and necessary daily tasks.

Developing effective routines for a child with ASD involves thoughtful planning and consideration of the child's needs, capabilities, and interests. Start by observing the times of day when your child is most receptive to engaging in various activities. Utilize these peak times for more demanding tasks such as educational activities or therapies. Simple, consistent morning and bedtime routines can help frame the day with a comfortable predictability. It's also beneficial to involve your child in the creation of these routines. This can be achieved by offering limited choices, such as deciding between two activities for a particular time slot or choosing between outfit options. Involving children in these decisions helps increase their engagement and compliance with the routine, as they feel a sense of ownership and control over their daily activities.

However, while consistency is key, it's equally important to cultivate some flexibility within these routines to handle unexpected changes without significant distress. For instance, if a particular activity in the routine gets disrupted, having a 'backup' option that's already familiar to the child can be helpful. Teaching children that sometimes activities might change, and modeling calm adjustment to these changes, can reduce anxiety associated with disruptions. This flexibility can be gradually introduced by initially making small changes in the routine and providing plenty of positive reinforcement for handling these changes well.

Using visual schedules can significantly aid in supporting routines for children with autism. Visual schedules use pictures to represent each activity planned for the day, providing a clear and accessible way for children to understand and anticipate what their day will involve. This can be particularly helpful for non-verbal or minimally verbal children, as it gives them a way to see their day without needing to rely solely on verbal explanations. These schedules should be placed in a common area where they are easily accessible to the child throughout the day, and parents should routinely refer to the schedule, guiding the child through each transition. As activities are completed, encouraging the child to remove or mark these activities on the schedule can also provide a sense of accomplishment and a clear visual cue that the activity is done, further reinforcing the structure provided by the routine.

By embedding routines into the daily lives of children with ASD, and using tools like visual schedules, parents can create a nurturing environment that fosters learning and development while reducing the stress associated with unpredictability. This structured approach not only supports the child's cognitive and emotional development but also enhances their ability to cope with the dynamic nature of everyday life, providing a solid foundation for growth and learning.

## 20.6 STRATEGIES FOR IMPROVING SLEEP IN CHILDREN WITH AUTISM

Sleep, a crucial pillar of health often taken for granted, can be a significant challenge for children with Autism Spectrum Disorder (ASD). Many parents find themselves navigating a maze of sleepless nights and erratic patterns that affect not only their child's well-being but the entire family's dynamics. Children with ASD may experience a range of sleep disturbances, including difficulty falling asleep, frequent awakenings during the night, and irregular sleep patterns that disrupt their ability to function optimally during daytime activities. These challenges are often compounded by heightened sensory sensitivities and difficulties in maintaining a sleep routine.

Good sleep hygiene practices are foundational to improving sleep quality in children with autism. Establishing a consistent bedtime routine is paramount. This routine might involve winding down activities an hour before bed, using calming techniques such as reading a story or listening to soft music, and ensuring the sleep environment is conducive to relaxation. The bedroom should be cool, quiet, and dark, and electronics should be removed to avoid stimulation from screens. For children with sensory sensitivities, the use of weighted blankets or blackout curtains can provide a sense of security and block out excess light and noise, creating a sanctuary that promotes easier transitions into sleep.

Addressing sleep hygiene is just the beginning. Behavioral interventions can also play a crucial role in managing sleep issues. Bedtime fading, which involves gradually adjusting bedtime to a later time to ensure the child is truly tired, can be effective. Over time, as the child begins to fall asleep more quickly, bedtime can be slowly moved back to a more desirable time. Sleep restriction methods, which limit the amount of time the child spends in bed awake, can also help consolidate sleep during the night. While these methods require consistency and patience, they often yield significant improvements in sleep quality and duration.

Positive reinforcements can further enhance these strategies. Rewarding the child for staying in bed or for not calling out after bedtime can reinforce good sleep habits. These rewards should be motivating and immediately follow the desired behavior to strengthen the association between the behavior and the positive outcome. A sticker chart or a small treat the next day can serve as effective motivational tools.

Despite best efforts with routines and behavioral strategies, some sleep issues may persist, necessitating professional intervention. Recognizing when to seek help is crucial. If sleep disturbances continue to impair the child's and family's daily life, it may be time to consult a healthcare provider. Professionals specializing in sleep disorders can offer guidance, and in some cases, may recommend further interventions such as melatonin supplements or a referral to a sleep specialist. Working with a healthcare provider can provide a tailored approach to address complex or persistent sleep problems, ensuring that your child receives the best possible care to meet their specific needs.

Navigating sleep challenges in children with ASD requires a multifaceted approach that incorporates good sleep hygiene, behavioral strategies, and, when necessary, professional guidance. By systematically addressing these aspects, you can help improve your child's sleep, which is essential for their overall health and well-being. As sleep patterns improve, you are likely to notice positive changes in mood, behavior, and daily functioning, reinforcing the importance of sleep in the holistic management of autism.

## 20.7 THE IMPACT OF FAMILY DYNAMICS ON AUTISM MANAGEMENT

Navigating the intricate landscape of family dynamics becomes particularly pivotal when managing Autism Spectrum Disorder (ASD). The family unit acts as the primary support system and significantly influences therapeutic outcomes and the overall well-being of a child with autism. Understanding the roles and interactions within a family can reveal how these relationships impact the management of autism, especially in relation to siblings, extended family members, and the marital or co-parenting relationship. Each member plays a distinct role, and the dynamics between them can either support or complicate the emotional and developmental progress of a child with ASD.

For siblings, the presence of a brother or sister with ASD can shape their childhood experiences, influencing everything from daily routines to family attention distribution. It's crucial for parents to foster an environment where siblings feel valued and included. Regular family meetings can serve as a platform where every member, including siblings, expresses their feelings and concerns openly. This practice not only acknowledges the siblings' experiences but also helps them understand the unique challenges faced by their brother or sister with autism, cultivating empathy and patience.

Equally, the division of responsibilities within the home needs careful consideration. Sharing responsibilities related to the care of a child with ASD can prevent caregiver burnout and ensure that no single family member feels overwhelmed. This approach also models teamwork and cooperation for all children in the family, providing them with a sense of security and stability. Furthermore, engaging in family activities that accommodate the interests and needs of all children can strengthen familial bonds and ensure that each member feels connected and significant.

In the broader context, extended family members such as grandparents or aunts and uncles can also play a supportive role in the network of care. Educating these family members about ASD and involving them in caregiving can extend the support system, providing respite for parents and different interactions for the child with ASD. However, it is essential to communicate effectively with extended family about the specific needs and behaviors associated with autism to ensure consistent and understanding care.

**Counseling and Family Therapy**

Considering the complexities involved, counseling or family therapy often becomes an invaluable resource in managing family dynamics when autism is part of the daily equation. Professional guidance can help resolve conflicts, improve communication, and strengthen the family unit by providing strategies tailored to the unique challenges of living with ASD. For instance, a therapist specialized in special needs can facilitate discussions that help family members understand each other's perspectives better, from the parents' challenges to the siblings' feelings of neglect or jealousy.

Therapy sessions can also address specific issues such as co-parenting strategies for parents who might struggle with differing views on how to best support their child with ASD. A neutral professional setting allows for open discussion of each parent's concerns and expectations, fostering a unified approach to parenting that is crucial for the child's consistent support.

Moreover, family therapy can equip members with practical tools to handle the stresses associated with ASD. Techniques such as stress management, crisis resolution, and proactive planning can be explored within therapy, providing families with skills that enhance their resilience and ability to work together effectively.

Through a better understanding of family dynamics, regular communication, shared responsibilities, and professional support, families can create a nurturing environment that not only supports the growth and development of the child with autism but also ensures the well-being of each family member. This holistic approach to autism management recognizes the interconnectedness of family relationships and the significant impact these relationships have on therapeutic outcomes. By fostering a supportive and understanding family environment, you lay a strong foundation for your child with ASD to thrive, ensuring that each family member is equipped to navigate the challenges and celebrate the successes together.

## 20.8 TRANSITIONING TO COLLEGE: PREPARING YOUR CHILD WITH AUTISM

The transition to college represents a significant milestone for any student, but for a young adult with Autism Spectrum Disorder (ASD), this step can entail unique challenges and opportunities. Preparing your child for college involves a multifaceted approach that begins with a thorough assessment of their readiness, extends to selecting the right college environment, and includes continuous support and advocacy to navigate college life successfully.

**College Readiness Assessment**

Assessing your child's readiness for college is the first crucial step in the transition process. This assessment should encompass several key areas: academic skills, social readiness, and daily living capabilities. Academically, evaluate whether your child has mastered the skills necessary to succeed in a more autonomous learning environment, including time management, study skills, and the ability to seek help when needed. Social readiness involves gauging your child's ability to manage interpersonal interactions, understand social norms, and develop relationships—skills that are essential for navigating the social dynamics of college life. Equally important are daily living skills such as laundry, budgeting, meal preparation, and transportation management, which are critical for students living away from home.

To conduct this assessment, consider consulting with your child's current educational team and possibly seeking evaluations from professionals who specialize in ASD. Together, you can develop a comprehensive profile of your child's strengths and areas where they might need further development or support. Use this information to create a targeted plan that addresses these needs, possibly through additional coursework, social skills training, or life skills coaching in the months leading up to college.

**Choosing the Right College**

Selecting an appropriate college is more than just looking at academic programs; it involves finding a campus that supports students with ASD both academically and socially. When evaluating potential colleges, look for institutions that offer specialized services for students with disabilities, such as tutoring, academic advising, counseling, and social clubs that promote inclusion. It's important to investigate the college's policies on accommodations and support services, ensuring they align with your child's needs.

Visiting campuses can be incredibly beneficial. During visits, meet with the disability services office to discuss specific accommodations your child might need, such as priority registration, note-taking services, or alternative testing arrangements. Also, consider the overall campus environment—everything from the physical layout to the student body's demeanor can impact how comfortable and supported your child will feel.

204 | AUTISM FOR PARENTS

## Preparation for College Life

Preparing your child for the realities of college life involves practical training and emotional support. Begin by fostering independence in daily living tasks, encouraging your child to take on more responsibilities at home. Simultaneously, help them develop a system to manage their schedule and commitments, which can include using digital tools like calendar apps or reminders. Social skills are also vital; consider enrolling your child in programs that simulate college social settings or provide opportunities for making friends and handling social interactions.

Discuss with your child the resources available on campus and how to access them. Knowing in advance where to go for help —be it academic support, counseling services, or health care— can alleviate much of the anxiety associated with new environments. Role-playing different scenarios, such as how to connect with professors or resolve conflicts with roommates, can also boost your child's confidence and preparedness.

## Continued Support and Advocacy

Even as your child takes on the new world of college, your role in providing support and advocacy remains crucial. Maintain regular communication with your child to monitor their well-being and academic progress. Encourage them to share their experiences, challenges, and successes, and be ready to step in with advice or intervention when necessary.

Advocating for your child may also involve ongoing communication with college staff and service providers to ensure that accommodations are being properly implemented and adjusted as needed. Teach your child self-advocacy skills so they can articulate their needs and rights, a crucial ability in college and beyond. Encouraging your child to join student advocacy groups or networks can also provide them with a platform to voice their needs and connect with peers facing similar challenges.

Preparing your child for college as a student with ASD involves thoughtful planning, proactive preparation, and ongoing support. By assessing readiness, choosing the right college environment, preparing for the demands of college life, and continuing to provide support and advocacy, you can help your child navigate this significant transition successfully. With the right tools and strategies, college can be a time of tremendous growth and achievement for your child, laying a foundation for future success in all areas of life.

## 20.9 ADULT DIAGNOSIS OF AUTISM: UNDERSTANDING AND COPING STRATEGIES

Receiving a diagnosis of Autism Spectrum Disorder (ASD) in adulthood can bring both clarity and a wave of new challenges. For many, this diagnosis comes after years of misunderstandings and misdiagnoses, offering an explanation for previous life struggles and differences. But it also raises complex questions about identity, relationships, and professional life. Let's explore how an adult diagnosis of autism can reshape an individual's understanding of themselves and their interactions with the world.

### Challenges and Benefits of a Late Diagnosis

An adult diagnosis often brings a profound sense of relief and validation. For years, you might have felt out of sync with your peers, struggling with social interactions or sensory sensitivities that didn't seem to affect others. Understanding that these experiences are due to ASD can lift a weight of self-blame and confusion. However, this revelation can also lead to a period of adjustment where you reassess past life events through a new lens, which can be emotionally taxing.

One of the pivotal challenges following a diagnosis is the potential shift in personal and professional relationships. Friends, family, or coworkers might not fully understand what autism entails, potentially leading to misunderstandings or changes in how they relate to you. It's crucial during this time to communicate openly about what your diagnosis means and doesn't mean, and how it affects your interactions and needs.

To illustrate, consider the story of Michael, a 35-year-old who was diagnosed with ASD at the age of 33. Prior to his diagnosis, he had difficulty maintaining relationships and employment, which led to significant stress and anxiety. After his diagnosis, with the support of a therapist, Michael began to understand his behavior patterns and sensory triggers better. He communicated his needs more effectively to those around him, leading to improved relationships and a more accommodating workplace.

## Navigating Post-Diagnosis Changes

Receiving an ASD diagnosis as an adult requires navigating significant life adjustments. These can include redefining personal identity, reshaping relationships, and making necessary changes in the workplace. It's important to approach these changes gradually and seek support from professionals who understand the implications of a late diagnosis.

For instance, you might need to establish new routines or modify your living environment to better suit sensory preferences that were previously unacknowledged. Professional life may also require adjustments; you might seek more structured tasks, clearer communication from supervisors, or even pursue a different career path that aligns more closely with your strengths and interests.

## Accessing Adult Autism Services

Post-diagnosis, it's vital to connect with services and supports tailored to adults with ASD. These can range from cognitive-behavioral therapy, which can help in developing coping strategies for anxiety and social interactions, to career counseling services that specialize in clients with ASD. Many communities offer support groups where you can meet others diagnosed in adulthood, providing a network of peers who understand the unique challenges you face.

Additionally, vocational programs designed for adults with ASD can offer training and employment opportunities in environments that recognize and accommodate neurodiver-

sity. These programs not only support professional development but also enhance social skills and community
integration.

### Emotional and Psychological Support

Adjusting to a late diagnosis of autism is not just about practical changes; it also involves managing emotional and
psychological impacts. Engaging with a therapist who
specializes in adult autism can provide a space to explore
feelings about the diagnosis and develop strategies for
managing anxiety and depression, which are common
among newly diagnosed adults.

Support groups play an essential role in providing emotional
and social support. These groups offer a platform to share
experiences, challenges, and successes with others who
understand the nuances of discovering one's neurodiversity
later in life. They can also be a source of information about
coping strategies and resources that others have found
helpful.

Living with an awareness of being on the autism spectrum
can bring a profound shift in how you view yourself and
navigate the world. While the initial adjustments post-diagnosis can be challenging, many find that understanding their
autism provides a framework for making life more accommodating to their needs. With the right support and strategies, the diagnosis of ASD in adulthood can lead to a deeper
understanding of oneself and a more authentic, fulfilling life.

## 20.10 AUTISM, AGING, AND LONG-TERM CARE PLANNING

As individuals with Autism Spectrum Disorder (ASD) advance in age, the landscape of their needs and support structures undergoes significant changes, necessitating a thoughtful approach to their long-term care. With aging comes potential shifts in cognitive function, physical health, and social needs, aspects that might not have been as pressing in the younger years. Understanding these evolving needs is crucial for ensuring that aging adults with autism continue to lead fulfilling and comfortable lives.

The aging process in autism can present unique challenges. Cognitive changes might include a decrease in the ability to process new information or maintain attention, which can affect daily functioning and independence. Physically, there may be an increased risk of co-occurring health issues such as epilepsy or sensory sensitivities that intensify with age. Socially, the support networks that were once robust may change as parents or caregivers age and siblings or peers move into different life stages. This shift can lead to a greater risk of isolation, making social engagement and community involvement even more vital.

Addressing these changes requires a proactive approach to long-term care planning. This planning should encompass a comprehensive evaluation of potential care needs, including medical, social, and daily living supports. It's also important to consider the living arrangements that will best support the individual's quality of life. Options might include specialized residential communities designed to accommodate adults with ASD, providing structured environments and

210 | AUTISM FOR PARENTS

community engagement activities that cater to their needs. In-home care services are another option, offering support in more familiar surroundings and allowing for a greater degree of continuity in daily routines.

Other considerations include adult day care programs, which can provide social opportunities and structured activities during the day, offering respite for caregivers and a stimulating environment for the individual. Each option has its benefits and considerations, and the choice will depend largely on the specific needs and preferences of the individual, as well as the resources available in their community.

**Planning for Future Care**

The task of planning for the future care of an adult with autism involves not only identifying the right care options but also ensuring that all legal and financial aspects are addressed. This includes establishing guardianships or trusts to protect the individual's interests and making sure that financial resources are in place to support long-term care needs. Creating a life care plan can serve as a roadmap, outlining the supports and services required throughout the individual's life and how these will be funded and provided.

Such planning should ideally involve legal and financial professionals who specialize in special needs planning. They can offer guidance on the best practices and tools for securing the future of an individual with ASD, ensuring that their rights are protected and their care is uninterrupted as they transition from one life stage to another.

## Support for Caregivers

Supporting the caregivers of aging adults with autism is equally important. Caregivers often face high levels of stress and burnout, especially as their loved ones' needs become more complex with aging. Providing them with access to resources and respite care services can help maintain their health and well-being, ensuring they can continue to provide support. This might include connecting them to support groups, educational resources to help them navigate the aging process in autism, and respite care options that allow them some much-needed downtime.

Community resources and health services can play a crucial role in supporting both individuals with autism and their caregivers. By fostering a supportive network and ensuring access to necessary services, caregivers can find the strength and assistance they need to manage the challenges that arise with aging and autism.

As we contemplate the future care of adults with autism, it becomes clear that comprehensive planning, community support, and adequate resources are essential for ensuring that they continue to live with dignity and quality. This proactive approach not only addresses the immediate needs but also sets a foundation for sustaining quality of life throughout the aging process. As we move forward, it is crucial that we continue to foster environments that respect and accommodate the unique needs of aging individuals with ASD, ensuring they remain integrated and active members of their communities.

# HELP OTHER PARENTS!

I hope you leave this book with a deeper level of understanding, feeling more confident about helping your child navigate life with ASD. Now you have a chance to help other parents too.

Simply by sharing your honest opinion of this book and a little about your own experience, you'll help new readers to connect with this resource, and, in turn, with their own child.

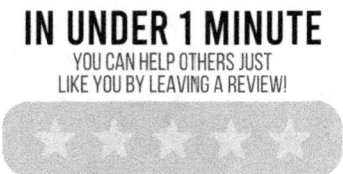

**IN UNDER 1 MINUTE**
YOU CAN HELP OTHERS JUST
LIKE YOU BY LEAVING A REVIEW!

Thank you so much for your support. You're making a powerful difference.

**Scan the QR code below**

# CONCLUSION

As we draw this guide to a close, it's important to reflect on the profound journey of understanding and acceptance that you, as a parent or caregiver, have embarked upon. From the initial whirlwind of diagnosis through the evolving stages of growth and challenge, your path is one of continuous learning and profound love. You are not just navigating a condition; you are embracing a whole unique person, advocating tirelessly for their needs and celebrating their distinct gifts.

This book has traversed the critical landscape of autism, starting with the pivotal role of early diagnosis. Recognizing the signs of autism early in a child's life opens doors to tailored interventions and therapies that can significantly influence their development and quality of life. We've explored personalized approaches to therapy and intervention that cater to individual needs, ensuring each child can thrive in their unique way.

The support of family and community stands as a pillar throughout this journey. As you have seen, building a nurturing and understanding environment involves everyone from siblings and extended family to teachers and fellow community members. The strength of these networks cannot be overstated—they are your allies, your support system, and often, your greatest advocates.

We've delved into the evolving landscape of autism research and treatment, highlighting the exciting advancements in genetic and neurological studies. The development of new technological aids for therapy and learning, alongside global efforts to better understand and treat autism, offer hope and practical help for addressing the challenges you and your child may face.

This book is also a call to action. It is an invitation to take your experiences and use them to fuel broader awareness and change. Advocate for more inclusive policies, educate your community, and help shift public perceptions about autism. Every conversation you start, every misconception you clear, contributes to a more accepting world.

As you move forward, remember that the field of autism is one of constant discovery. Stay open and adaptable to new information and strategies. What works today may evolve tomorrow, and staying informed is key to continuing to provide the best support for your child.

I urge you to take proactive steps to build a more inclusive society. Engage with local schools, workplaces, and policy-makers to create environments where individuals with autism are not just accommodated but truly valued for their unique perspectives and abilities.

Finally, let me leave you with words of hope and encouragement. The road may be challenging, but it is also filled with moments of joy and triumph. Your child has the potential to lead a fulfilling life, rich with achievements and happiness, supported by those who care and advocate alongside them.

As immediate next steps, consider reaching out to a local support group, checking online for the latest in autism research, or simply starting a dialogue about autism awareness in your community. Each step, no matter how small, is a stride toward greater understanding and inclusivity.

Remember, while this book provides a comprehensive guide, the journey with autism is deeply personal and unique to each family. Embrace the journey with patience, love, and the knowledge that you are making an incredible difference in your child's life.

Thank you for allowing me to be a part of your journey. Together, let's continue to learn, to support, and to advocate for a world where every individual with autism is recognized not just for their challenges, but for their incredible potential to enrich our lives and communities.....and finally while the corpus of this book has ended, please review all the references below as they represent a virtual cornucopia of references and links that will give you a lot more detail than what we had space and time to provide above. Enjoy and thank you !!!!

# REFERENCES

DSM-5TR Updates Autism Diagnostic Criteria
https://www.wpspublish.com/blog/dsm-5tr-
updates-autism-diagnostic-criteria

Early Intervention for Autism | NICHD https://
www.nichd.nih.gov/health/topics/autism/
conditioninfo/treatments/early-intervention

Co-Occurring Conditions and Autism https://
autism.org/comorbidities-of-autism/

Racial/Ethnic Disparities in the Identification of
Children ... https://www.ncbi.nlm.nih.gov/
pmc/articles/PMC2661453/

Early Intervention for Autism | NICHD https://
www.nichd.nih.gov/health/topics/autism/
conditioninfo/treatments/early-intervention

Siblings of autistic children and teenagers
https://raisingchildren.net.au/autism/commu
nicating-relationships/family-relationships/
siblings-asd

Archived: Guide to the Individualized Education
Program        https://www2.ed.gov/parents/
needs/speced/iepguide/index.html

Support for family members https://www.autism
speaks.org/autism-support-family-help

Visual Supports and Autism Spectrum Disorders
https://vkc.vumc.org/assets/files/resources/
visualsupports.pdf

The Best Free Apps for Nonverbal Autism https://getgoally.com/blog/5-free-apps-for-nonverbal-autism/

15 Speech Therapy Exercises for Children with Autism https://stamurai.com/blog/speech-therapy-exercises-for-children-with-autism/

Understanding Nonverbal Autism https://www.verywellhealth.com/what-is-nonverbal-autism-260032

Here's Why an Autism Routine is Important https://www.autismparentingmagazine.com/autism-routine-importance/

Sensory-Friendly Home Modifications for Autism https://www.turbotenant.com/blog/home-modifications-for-autism/

What is a Sensory Diet for Autism? https://www.
autismparentingmagazine.com/sensory-diet-
for-autism/

Top 5 autism tips: managing sensory differences
https://www.autism.org.uk/advice-and-guid
ance/professional-practice/sensory-differ
ences

Guide to Individualized Education Programs
(IEP)       https://www.autismspeaks.org/tool-
kit/guide-individualized-education-
programs-iep

The Benefits of Inclusion for Students on the
Autism      Spectrum      https://eric.ed.gov/?
id=EJ1304391

Parents' Experiences in Advocating for Children
and Youth ... https://www.ncbi.nlm.nih.gov/
pmc/articles/PMC8883377/

Assistive Technology for Students with Autism Spectrum ... https://www.naset.org/filead min/user_u pload/Autism_Series/Assist_tech/ AssistiveTech_for_Students_W_Autism.pdf

Supporting Play in Early Childhood: Specific Strategies for ... https://blog.stageslearning. com/blog/supporting-play-in-early-child hood-specific-strategies-for-children-with-autism

Choosing the best toys for children with ASD or ID https://www.miriamfoundation.ca/en/ whats-new/42-choosing-the-best-toys-for-children-with-asd-or-id.html

Making (and Keeping) Friends: A Model for Social Skills ... https://iidc.indiana.edu/irca/ articles/making-and-keeping-friends.html

Strategies in supporting inclusive education for autistic ... https://www.ncbi.nlm.nih.gov/ pmc/articles/PMC9620685/

Understanding Challenging Behaviors in Autism Spectrum ... https://www.ncbi.nlm.nih.gov/pmc/articles/PMC9324526/

What causes autism? Genetic and environmental factors https://www.medicalnewstoday.com/articles/what-causes-autism

Positive Behavioral Interventions and Supports https://autismspectrumnews.org/positive-behavioral-interventions-and-supports-an-effective-approach-for-schools-to-prevent-and-manage-challenging-behaviors/

Functional Behavioral Assessment for Children with Autism https://www.autismparenting magazine.com/autism-functional-behavioral-assessment/

Top 10 AAC (Augmentative & Alternative Communication ... https://www.speechpathol ogygraduateprograms.org/2017/11/top-10-aac-augmentative-and-alternative-communi cation-devices/

Assistive Technology for Autism: Tools and Benefits https://www.verywellhealth.com/assistive-technology-for-autism-5076159

Best Apps for Autism: 12 Apps for Development and Skill- ... https://www.hopebridge.com/blog/best-apps-for-autism/

The Impact of Technology on People with Autism Spectrum ... https://www.ncbi.nlm.nih.gov/pmc/articles/PMC6832622/

Multi-level analysis of the gut–brain axis shows autism ... https://www.nature.com/articles/s41593-023-01361-0

A systematic review and meta-analysis of the benefits ... https://pubmed.ncbi.nlm.nih.gov/34617108/

Autism and Exercise: Special Benefits https://
www.autismspeaks.org/expert-opinion/
autism-exercise-benefits

15 Speech Therapy Exercises for Children with
Autism      https://autismcenterforkids.com/
speech-therapy-exercises/

Supporting Mental Health in Children with
Autism    https://scsmh.education.uiowa.edu/
2023/04/04/supporting-mental-health-in-
children-with-autism/

Self-Care Tips for Parents of Special Needs
Children https://www.goodtherapy.org/blog/
self-care-tips-for-parents-of-special-needs-
children-0810175/

Cognitive Behavioral Therapy and Autism
Spectrum    ...    https://www.kennedykrieger.
org/stories/interactive-autism-network-ian/
cognitive_behavioral_therapy

Autism and Puberty - Child Mind Institute https://childmind.org/article/autism-and-puberty/

Sex Education and Autism https://sparkforautism.org/discover_article/sex-education-and-autism/

Life Skills and Autism https://www.autismspeaks.org/life-skills-and-autism

Transition to Adulthood - Autism Speaks https://www.autismspeaks.org/transition-adulthood

Vocational Training For Adults With Autism https://adultautismcenter.org/programs/vocational-training-for-adults-with-autism/

Essential Life Skills for Adults with Autism https://www.romanempireagency.com/blog/autism/essential-life-skills-for-adults-with-autism/

Employment Rights | Autism Speaks https://www.autismspeaks.org/tool-kit-excerpt/employment-rights

Social Skills and Autism https://www.autismspeaks.org/social-skills-and-autism

Understanding the Differences Between IDEA and Section 504 https://www.ldonline.org/ld-topics/special-education/understanding-differences-between-idea-and-section-504

Health Care Rights for Autistic Patients https://adult-autism.health.harvard.edu/resources/health-care-rights-for-autistic-patients/

Individuals With Autism Spectrum Disorder and
Employment    https://adata.org/legal_brief/
autism-spectrum-disorder-and-employment

Parents' Experiences in Advocating for Children
and Youth ... https://www.ncbi.nlm.nih.gov/
pmc/articles/PMC8883377/

Starting    an    Autism    Support/Self-Advocacy
Group            https://paautism.org/resource/
support-self-advocacy-group/

Understanding the Implications of Peer Support
for ... https://www.ncbi.nlm.nih.gov/pmc/arti
cles/PMC8649771/

Finding Your Community https://www.autisms
peaks.org/finding-your-community

Autism Society Creating connections for the Autism community ... https://autismsociety.org/

Influence of Community-Level Cultural Beliefs about ... https://www.ncbi.nlm.nih.gov/pmc/articles/PMC7008392/

Understanding Stigma in Autism: A Narrative Review and ... https://www.ncbi.nlm.nih.gov/pmc/articles/PMC8992913/

Complementary and Alternative Therapies for Autism ... https://www.ncbi.nlm.nih.gov/pmc/articles/PMC4439475/

In Search of Culturally Appropriate Autism Interventions https://www.ncbi.nlm.nih.gov/pmc/articles/PMC5889961/

20 Famous People With Autism Spectrum Disorder (ASD) https://behavioral-innovations.com/blog/20-famous-people-with-autism-spectrum-disorder-asd/

Study Finds Early Intervention Highly Effective https://www.autismspeaks.org/science-news/early-intervention-toddlers-autism-highly-effective-study-finds

Helping Your Child with Autism Thrive https://www.helpguide.org/articles/autism-learning-disabilities/helping-your-child-with-autism-thrive.htm

Navigating the Education System with Autism https://www.lrcss.com/navigating-the-education-system

Associations Between Conceptual Reasoning, Problem ... https://www.ncbi.nlm.nih.gov/pmc/articles/PMC6067678/

Investigating a Multimodal Intervention for Children With ... https://www.ncbi.nlm.nih.gov/pmc/articles/PMC4619181/

Three Strategies to Strengthen Communication for Adults with Autism and Learning Differences https://autismspectrumnews.org/three-strategies-to-strengthen-communication-for-adults-with-autism-and-learning-differences/

Evidence-Based Practices for Children, Youth, and Young ... https://www.ncbi.nlm.nih.gov/pmc/articles/PMC8510990/

Kevin's Progress: An ABA Success Story - Circle Care Services https://circlecareservices.com/kevins-progress-another-aba-success-story/

Autism Care: The Role of the Family-Centered Care Team https://www.totalcareaba.com/autism/family-centered-autism-care-team

New genetic clues uncovered in largest study of families ... https://www.uclahealth.org/news/ release/new-genetic-clues-uncovered-largest-study-families-with

Early Autism Screening: A Comprehensive Review - PMC https://www.ncbi.nlm.nih. gov/pmc/articles/PMC6765988/

The Impact of Technology on People with Autism Spectrum ... https://www.ncbi.nlm. nih.gov/pmc/articles/PMC6832622/

The International Collaboration for Autism Registry Epidemiology (iCARE) - NCBI https://www.ncbi.nlm.nih.gov/pmc/arti cles/PMC4512211/

Sharing an Autism Diagnosis With Family and Friends https://childmind.org/article/shar ing-an-autism-diagnosis-with-family-and-friends/

Success Stories of Individuals with Autism - Healing Haven https://thehealinghaven.net/success-stories-of-individuals-with-autism/

Strategies for Managing Anxiety in Children With Autism https://premierpediatrictherapy.com/blog/strategies-for-managing-anxiety-in-children-with-autism/

"80 Autism Quotes to Inspire and Educate." Apex ABA Therapy | A World Of Smiles. A Life Of Fulfillment. Last modified June 13, 2024. https://www.apexaba.com/blog/autism-quotes

www.ingramcontent.com/pod-product-compliance
Lightning Source LLC
Chambersburg PA
CBHW061733120626
46550CB00005B/1784

* 9 7 9 8 2 1 8 5 8 7 0 7 9 *